Strategies for
Alternate
Item Formats
on the NCLEX-RN® Exam

Strategies for
Alternate
Item Formats
on the NCLEX-RN® Exam

Linda Anne Silvestri, MSN, RN
Instructor of Nursing
Salve Regina University
Newport, Rhode Island
President
Nursing Reviews, Inc.
and
Professional Nursing Seminars, Inc.
Charlestown, Rhode Island
Instructor of NCLEX-RN® and NCLEX-PN®
    Review Courses

Yazmin Mojica, MSN/MPH, MA, RN, CNS
Instructor of NCLEX-RN® and NCLEX-PN®
    Test Preparation
Nursing Education Consultant
President
National NCLEX® Solutions
and
MYEC™ Education and Consulting Services
Walnut, California

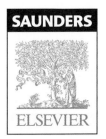

SAUNDERS

ELSEVIER

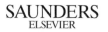

SAUNDERS
ELSEVIER

11830 Westline Industrial Drive
St. Louis, Missouri 63146

STRATEGIES FOR ALTERNATE ITEM FORMATS   ISBN: 978-1-4160-3841-2
ON THE NCLEX-RN® EXAM

NCLEX and NCLEX-RN® are registered trademarks and service marks of the National Council of State Boards of Nursing, Inc.

ISBN: 978-1-4160-3841-2

Managing Editor: Nancy O'Brien
Developmental Editor: Charlene R.M. Ketchum
Publishing Services Manager: Deborah L. Vogel
Senior Project Manager: Deon Lee
Multimedia Producer: Amy Shehi
Senior Book Designer: Amy Buxton

Printed in United States of America

Last digit is the print number: 9   8   7   6   5   4   3   2   1

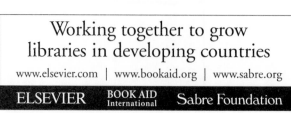

To all nursing students—
Your passion to help those in need is the greatest gift that
you can give to the profession.
We wish you continued success throughout your nursing program and in
your new career as a Registered Nurse!

Linda and Yazmin

About the Authors

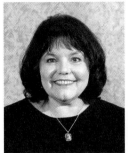

Photo by Laurent W. Valliere

Linda Anne Silvestri received her diploma in nursing at Cooley Dickinson Hospital School of Nursing in Northampton, Massachusetts. She later received an Associate's degree from Holyoke Community College in Holyoke, Massachusetts, and then received her BSN from American International College in Springfield, Massachusetts. In 1985, Linda earned her MSN from Anna Maria College, Paxton, Massachusetts, with a dual major in Nursing Management and Patient Education, and presently she is attending the University of Nevada to earn a PhD in Nursing.

Linda is a nursing instructor at Salve Regina University. She is also a member of Sigma Theta Tau and the President of Nursing Reviews, Inc., and Professional Nursing Seminars, Inc. Linda has been conducting NCLEX-RN® and NCLEX-PN® review courses throughout New England since 1991 to assist nursing graduates to achieve their goals of becoming Registered Nurses and/or Licensed Practical/Vocational Nurses.

Linda is the successful author of numerous NCLEX-RN and NCLEX-PN review products, including *Saunders Comprehensive Review for the NCLEX-RN® Examination, Saunders Q & A Review for the NCLEX-RN® Examination, Saunders Strategies for Success for the NCLEX-RN® Examination, Saunders Comprehensive Review for the NCLEX-PN® Examination, Saunders Q & A Review for the NCLEX-PN® Examination, Saunders Strategies for Success for the NCLEX-PN® Examination, Saunders Review Cards for the NCLEX-PN® Examination,* and *Saunders Instructor's Resource Package for NCLEX-PN®*. Linda has also authored the *Saunders Online Review Course for the NCLEX-RN® Examination*.

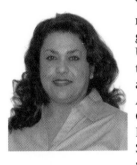

Yazmin Mojica began her nursing career in 1981 after graduating from the Los Angeles Unified School District's Vocational Nursing Program located at Jordan Locke Community Adult School in Los Angeles, California. She then attended Rancho Santiago College in Santa Ana California, where she completed the Registered Nursing Program in 1988 and received an Associate's degree in Nursing. In 1996, Yazmin received a Bachelor of Science degree in Nursing from California State University, Fullerton. She continued her education and in 2000 earned a Master of Arts degree in Occupational Studies/Vocational Education. In 2003, she graduated with honors, Phi Kappa Phi, when she received a dual Master's degree in Nursing and Public Health from California State University, Long Beach.

Yazmin is a Clinical Nurse Specialist in Program Development, Assessment, and Evaluation; a book chapter author in critical thinking; a Genome Scholar from the National Institutes of Health; an Honorary Member of Sigma Theta Tau; and a Continuing Education Provider for Registered Nurses. Yazmin has taught both practical/vocational and registered nursing students. Currently she is the president of National NCLEX® Solutions and MYEC™ Education and Consulting Services. Yazmin has developed several NCLEX-PN and NCLEX-RN test preparation and review courses and travels throughout the state of California presenting these courses. Additionally, Yazmin works as an education consultant in nursing schools and a variety of health care organizations throughout California.

Faculty and Student Reviewers

▲▲▲

Faculty Reviewers

Cynthia Dakin, PhD, RN
Assistant Professor
Northeastern University, School of Nursing
Boston, Massachusetts

Brenda Sloan, RN, MA, APRN, BC
Assistant Professor
Indiana Wesleyan University, Department of Nursing
Marion, Indiana

Donna Walls, BS, MS
Assistant Clinical Professor
Texas Women's University, College of Nursing
Dallas, Texas

Student Reviewers

Monika Bixler
Lebanon County Career and Technology Center
Lebanon, Pennsylvania

Jocelyn Hoffman
Northeastern University
Boston, Massachusetts

Courtney Leach
Northeastern University
Boston, Massachusetts

Preface

▲▲▲

Welcome to *Saunders Pyramid to Success*!

Strategies for Alternate Item Formats for the NCLEX-RN® Exam is one component in a series of products designed to assist you in achieving your goal of becoming a registered nurse and is a companion text to all of the other products in *Saunders Pyramid to Success* for the NCLEX-RN examination. It differs from other products in the *Saunders Pyramid to Success* in that it contains *ONLY* alternate item format questions. These alternate item format questions include fill-in-the-blank, multiple response, prioritizing (ordered response), figure/illustration (hot spot), and chart/exhibit questions. This book provides you with all of the information that you need to correctly answer all types of alternate item format questions that may appear on your nursing examinations and on the NCLEX-RN examination.

ORGANIZATION OF THE BOOK

Strategies for Alternate Item Formats for the NCLEX-RN® Exam contains five chapters and a Comprehensive Test. Chapter 1 identifies test-taking strategies for each type of alternate item format question. Chapters 2 through 5 are specifically designed to address each Client Needs category of the NCLEX-RN Test Plan. These Client Needs categories include Safe and Effective Care Environment (Chapter 2), Health Promotion and Maintenance (Chapter 3), Psychosocial Integrity (Chapter 4), and Physiological Integrity (Chapter 5). Each of these chapters provides practice alternate item format questions specific to the Client Needs category addressed in the chapter. The Comprehensive Test provides practice alternate item format questions representative of all Client Needs categories.

The book contains 265 practice alternate item format questions. The accompanying CD contains the 265 practice alternate item format questions from the book and 15 additional questions with sound components that test your nursing knowledge about heart and lung sounds, for a total of 280 questions on the CD. All of the practice questions are reflective of the framework and the content identified in the current NCLEX-RN test plan. In addition to the Client Needs category, each practice question identifies a Level of Cognitive Ability, an Integrated Process (Caring, Communication and Documentation, Nursing Process step, or Teaching and Learning), and a content area based on designated subcategories of the Client Needs categories.

Chapter 1: Test-Taking Strategies for Alternate Item Format Questions

This chapter describes the various types of alternate item format questions that you may encounter on the NCLEX-RN examination and on the nursing examinations that you take during your nursing program. These alternate item format questions include the following: fill-in-the-blank, multiple response, prioritizing (ordered response), figure/illustration (hot spot), and chart/exhibit questions. Sample questions are provided for each type of alternate item format, along with specific test-taking strategies for answering correctly.

Chapter 2: Safe and Effective Care Environment Questions

The Safe and Effective Care Environment category constitutes 21% to 33% of the NCLEX-RN examination. This chapter provides specific information about this Client Needs category and its content areas and contains 45 alternate item format questions that specifically address Safe and Effective Care Environment. All types of alternate item formats are presented. Nursing content areas for these practice questions are coded as either *Management of Care* or *Safety and Infection Control*.

Chapter 3: Health Promotion and Maintenance Questions

The Health Promotion and Maintenance category constitutes 6% to 12% of the NCLEX-RN examination. This chapter contains 20 alternate item format questions that specifically address this Client Needs category. All types of alternate item formats are presented. This chapter also provides a description of this Client Needs category and identifies the content that is tested in this category. Nursing content areas for these practice questions are coded as either *Growth and Transitions Across the Life Span* or *Prevention and Detection of Health Alterations*.

Chapter 4: Psychosocial Integrity Questions

The Psychosocial Integrity category constitutes 6% to 12% of the NCLEX-RN® examination. This chapter provides a description of this Client Needs category and identifies the content that is tested in this category. Included in this chapter are 20 alternate item format questions that specifically address Psychosocial Integrity content areas. Nursing content areas for these practice questions are coded as either *Psychosocial Adaptation* or *Mental Health Disorders*.

Chapter 5: Physiological Integrity Questions

The Physiological Integrity category constitutes 43% to 67% of the NCLEX-RN examination. There are 105 alternate item format questions in this chapter, and these questions specifically address the Client Needs category Physiological Integrity. All types of alternate item formats are presented. This chapter also provides a description of this Client Needs category and identifies the content that is tested in each subcategory. Nursing content areas for these practice questions are coded as *Basic Care and Comfort, Pharmacological and Parenteral Therapies, Reduction of Risk Potential,* or *Physiological Adaptation*.

Comprehensive Test

The Comprehensive Test contains 75 alternate item format questions representative of all Client Needs categories of the NCLEX-RN test plan. All types of alternate item formats are presented in this section.

SPECIAL FEATURES OF THE BOOK
Practice Test Questions

Chapters 2 through 5 and the Comprehensive Test contain 265 practice questions in the alternate item formats. Each practice question provides a specific test-taking strategy that assists in answering the question correctly. The CD that accompanies the book contains the 265 practice questions located in the book plus an additional 15 questions with sound components that test your nursing knowledge of heart and lung sounds. There are 280 practice test questions on the CD.

Alternate Item Format Practice Test Questions

The alternate item format questions included in this book include fill-in-the-blank, multiple response, prioritizing (ordered response), figure/illustration (hot spot), and chart/exhibit questions. Additionally, the CD that accompanies this book contains both heart and lung sound questions.

Answer Section for Practice Test Questions

The answer sections for each practice test question in the book and on the accompanying CD include the correct answer, rationale, test-taking strategy, question categories, and reference source. The structure for the answer section is unique and provides the following information.

Rationale: The rationale provides you with the significant information regarding both correct and incorrect options.

Test-Taking Strategy: The test-taking strategy provides you with the logical path in selecting the correct answer and assists you in selecting an answer to a question on which you must guess. Specific suggestions for review are identified in the test-taking strategy.

Question Categories: Each question is identified based on the categories used by the NCLEX-RN test plan. Additional content area categories, designed to identify subcategories of each Client Needs areas, are provided with each question. The categories identified with each practice question include Level of Cognitive Ability, Client Needs, Integrated Process, and the designated subcategory area (content area). All categories are identified by their full names, so that you do not need to memorize codes or abbreviations.

Reference: A reference, including a page number, is provided so you can easily find the information that you need to review in major Elsevier textbooks.

NCLEX-RN Review CD

Packaged in this book is a CD that contains 280 alternate item format practice questions. These include fill-in-the-blank, multiple response, prioritizing (ordered response), figure/illustration, and chart/exhibit questions, as well as questions with heart and lung sound components. In addition to audio components, the CD utilizes a "drag and drop" capability for prioritizing (ordered response) questions, a "point and click" capability for figure/illustration and chart/exhibit questions, and a drop-down calculator for questions requiring calculation. This Windows- and Macintosh-compatible CD offers two testing modes for review.

Study: In this mode, students may review their results immediately after answering each practice question. These results include the answer, rationale, test-taking strategy, question categories, and reference source.

Examination: In this mode the student receives 50 randomly chosen questions from the entire pool of 280 questions. The answer, rationale, test-taking strategy, question categories, reference source, and results appear after you answer all 50 questions.

Selection Areas on the CD

When you use the CD, you will be able to select practice questions based on a Client Needs area, designated subcategory area (Content Area), category of Integrated Process, or alternate item format question type. These specific areas are identified below.

Client Needs Areas

Safe and Effective Care Environment
Health Promotion and Maintenance
Physiological Integrity
Psychosocial Integrity

Subcategory Area (Content Area)

Management of Care
Safety and Infection Control
Growth and Transitions Across the Life Span
Prevention and Detection of Health Alterations
Psychosocial Adaptation
Mental Health Disorders
Basic Care and Comfort
Pharmacological and Parenteral Therapies
Reduction of Risk Potential
Physiological Adaptation

Category of Integrated Process

Caring
Communication and Documentation
Nursing Process (Assessment, Analysis, Planning, Implementation, Evaluation)
Teaching and Learning

Alternate Item Format Question Type

Fill in the blank
Multiple response
Prioritizing (ordered response)
Figure/illustration (hot spot)
Chart/exhibit
Heart and lung sounds

HOW TO USE THIS BOOK

Strategies for Alternate Item Formats on the NCLEX-RN Exam® is especially designed to help you with your successful journey to the peak of the *Saunders Pyramid to Success*—becoming a registered nurse. This book focuses on alternate item format questions and the test-taking strategies for answering these types of questions. Alternate item format questions appear on the NCLEX-RN examination and on the nursing examinations that you take during your nursing program. It is critically important that you become familiar with these question types and the strategies for answering them correctly in order to relieve anxiety related to test taking and to achieve success in nursing examinations and in the NCLEX examination.

You should begin your process through this book by reading Chapter 1 because this chapter describes each type of alternate item format question and its accompanying specific test-taking strategy. Next, proceed through each chapter and read each practice question. Once you have answered a practice test question, read the rationale and the test-taking strategy. The rationale provides you with the significant information regarding both the correct and incorrect options. The test-taking strategy offers you the logical path to selecting the correct option. The strategy also identifies content area that you need to review if you had difficulty with the question. Use the reference source listed to easily find the information that you need to review. Finally, use the CD that accompanies this book and answer the practice questions. This will strengthen your knowledge base and skills in answering these types of questions and at the same time simulate the computer experience needed for taking the NCLEX-RN examination.

When using the CD, it is best to begin by selecting the Study Mode because you will receive immediate feedback regarding the answer, rationale, test-taking strategy, question codes, and reference source. Therefore you are provided with immediate information about your strengths and weaknesses.

It is important to identify your strengths and weaknesses. Additionally, it is important to strengthen any weak areas in order to be successful on the NCLEX-RN examination. Several other products in *Saunders Pyramid to Success* can be used to strengthen any weak areas. These additional products are described in Chapter 1 under the heading "What Are the Accompanying Products in *Saunders Pyramid to Success* for the NCLEX-RN® Examination?"

These products also can be obtained by calling 800-426-4545 or visiting www.elsevierhealth.com.

We wish you the very best with your journey through the *Saunders Pyramid to Success* and know that your hard work, perseverance, and self-confidence will bring you success in every journey that you take!

Linda Anne Silvestri, MSN, RN
Yazmin Mojica, MSN/MPH, MA, RN, CNS

Acknowledgments ▲▲▲

There are so many individuals who in their own way have contributed to the publication of this book. Our sincere appreciation and warmest thanks are extended to all of them.

First, we sincerely acknowledge and thank two very special and important individuals from Elsevier. We thank Nancy O'Brien, Managing Editor, for all of her assistance and ideas with creating this publication. We also thank Charlene Ketchum, Developmental Editor, for her expert organization skills, for maintaining order for all of the work that we submitted for manuscript production, and for her tremendous support during the entire preparation and production process. We especially want to acknowledge both Nancy and Charlene for their support of our ideas to create this product.

We also want to acknowledge all of the staff at Elsevier Health Sciences for their tremendous assistance throughout the preparation and production of this publication. We thank all of the special people in the Production Department, Debbie Vogel, Publication Services Manager; Deon Lee, Senior Project Manager; Amy Shehi, Multimedia Producer; and Amy Buxton, Senior Book Designer, whose expertise assisted in finalizing this publication.

We sincerely thank Bob Boehringer, Director of Nursing Marketing, and Andrew Eilers, former Marketing Manager, whose support, hard work, and special creativity assisted with this publication.

We also want to acknowledge Patricia Mieg, Educational Sales Representative for Elsevier Health Sciences, and Jeffrey S. Leber, Senior Account Manager, Special Markets for Elsevier Health Sciences, for their continuous encouragement and support.

Lastly, we want to thank all of our nursing students, past, present, and future, because their enthusiasm and aspiration to learn have inspired us to pursue our professional dreams.

A very sincere and special thank you to all of you!

Linda Anne Silvestri, MSN, RN
Yazmin Mojica, MSN/MPH, MA, RN, CNS

Contents

▲ ▲ ▲

1 *Test-Taking Strategies for Alternate Item Format Questions,* 1

2 *Safe and Effective Care Environment Questions,* 13

3 *Health Promotion and Maintenance Questions,* 63

4 *Psychosocial Integrity Questions,* 87

5 *Physiological Integrity Questions,* 111

Comprehensive Test, 221

Test-Taking Strategies for Alternate Item Format Questions

An important strategy for success during your nursing program and for the National Council Licensure Examination (NCLEX-RN®) is to become as familiar as possible with the types of questions that may appear in these examinations. A significant amount of anxiety can occur in a test-taker facing the challenge of nursing examinations. Knowing what the examination is all about will assist in alleviating your fear and anxiety.

This chapter describes the various types of alternate item format questions that you may encounter on the NCLEX-RN examination and on the nursing examinations that you take during your nursing program. It provides you with test-taking strategies to answer them correctly.

Why Is This an Essential Resource?

Alternate item format questions are questions that are designed to test your competency with regard to nursing skills and abilities. You may encounter these types of questions not only on the NCLEX-RN examination but also on the nursing examinations you take during your nursing program. Therefore, to achieve success both during your nursing education and on the NCLEX-RN examination, it is critical to be familiar with these types of questions and the test-taking strategies for answering them correctly.

This resource is one of a series of products designed to assist you in achieving your goal of becoming a registered nurse and is a companion text to all the other products in *Saunders Pyramid to Success for the NCLEX-RN® Examination*. It differs from all the other products in that it contains *only* alternate item format questions. It provides you with all the information you need about all types of alternate item format questions that may appear on your nursing examinations and on the NCLEX-RN examination. It contains 265 practice alternate item format questions and heart and lung sounds questions to prepare you for your nursing examinations and that most important examination, the NCLEX-RN. This chapter also provides information about all of the accompanying products in the *Saunders Pyramid to Success for the NCLEX-RN® Examination*. Remember, to alleviate anxiety and fear related to nursing examinations

and the NCLEX-RN examination and to be successful, it is critical for you to be as prepared as you can possibly be.

How Does This Resource Relate to the NCLEX-RN® Test Plan?

The content of NCLEX-RN reflects the activities that a newly licensed entry-level registered nurse must be able to perform to provide clients with safe and effective nursing care. The framework or Test Plan for the NCLEX-RN is based on Client Needs (Box 1-1). The chapters in this resource are organized based on these Client Needs. The NCLEX-RN Test Plan also indicates the incorporation of Integrated Processes throughout the Client Needs areas (Box 1-2). Therefore each alternate item format question in this book identifies its associated Client Needs area and Integrated Process. Additionally, the codes accompanying each question also identify the Level of Cognitive Ability, or difficulty level. Additional information about the components of the NCLEX-RN Test Plan and examination itself can be obtained by contacting the National Council of State Boards of Nursing (NCSBN) (Box 1-3).

What Are Alternate Item Format Questions?

Alternate item format questions are examination questions that may not include a multiple-choice format. These types of questions include fill-in-the-blanks, multiple-response questions, prioritizing (ordered response) questions, questions that contain a figure or illustration, and chart/exhibit questions (Box 1-4). Some alternate item format questions, such as the

BOX 1-2 ▲ INTEGRATED PROCESSES

- Caring
- Communication and Documentation
- Nursing Process
- Teaching and Learning

BOX 1-3 ▲ NATIONAL COUNCIL OF STATE BOARDS OF NURSING CONTACT INFORMATION

111 E. Wacker Drive
Suite 2900
Chicago, IL 60601
(312) 525-3600
www.ncsbn.org

BOX 1-1 ▲ CLIENT NEEDS

- Safe and Effective Care Environment
- Health Promotion and Maintenance
- Psychosocial Integrity
- Physiological Integrity

BOX 1-4 ▲ ALTERNATE ITEM FORMAT QUESTION TYPES

- Fill-in-the-blank
- Multiple response
- Prioritizing (ordered response/drag and drop)
- Figure/illustration (hot spots)
- Chart/exhibit

BOX 1-5 ▲ TEST-TAKING STRATEGIES: FILL-IN-THE-BLANK

- Always follow the directions on the computer screen.
- Use the erasable noteboard to perform the calculation.
- Read the question, set up the formula, and place the data from the question into the formula to solve the problem.
- Be alert to the need to perform conversions.
- Perform the calculation.
- Verify your answer using the on-screen calculator.
- Round answer to the nearest tenth or to a whole number if asked to do so.
- Place a zero before a decimal point and avoid placing trailing zeroes following the decimal point in the answer.

fill-in-the-blanks, may require that you use the computer keyboard to type in a numerical answer. Other alternate item format questions, such as the multiple response, those that present a figure or illustration, prioritizing (ordered response), and chart/exhibit questions, may require you to use the computer mouse to answer the question. In a multiple-response question you may need to use the computer mouse to click in a small box that indicates the correct answer(s). In a figure/illustration question, you may be asked to "point and click" (using the mouse) on a specific area (represented by a circle and also known as the "hot spot"). For example, you may be presented with a figure that displays the thorax of an adult client and may be asked to "point and click" at the area where vesicular breath sounds are auscultated. In a prioritizing (ordered response) question, you may be asked to use the computer mouse and to "drag and drop" the answers presented in order of priority. In a chart/exhibit question you need to use the computer mouse to click on designated exhibit buttons and tab buttons to read the information in order to answer the question.

NCSBN provides specific directions for you to follow with these questions to guide you in your testing process. It is very important to read these directions as they appear on the computer screen. NCSBN also provides a tutorial at the start of the examination to assist you in answering these types of questions. However, by using this resource, you will already be familiar with these question types, so this will save you time during testing and of course will relieve some anxiety. We also encourage you to access the NCSBN website at www.ncsbn.org and Pearson VUE website at www.pearsonvue.com/nclex to obtain additional information about the NCLEX-RN examination and these types of questions, and to review the tutorial that the NCSBN provides for you.

WHAT TEST-TAKING STRATEGIES ARE HELPFUL FOR ANSWERING FILL-IN-THE-BLANK QUESTIONS?

Fill-in-the-blank questions ask you to perform a medication calculation, calculate an intravenous flow rate or infusion time for a specific intravenous solution, or calculate an intake or output record on a client. You need to type in your answer, which will be in a numerical format. In other words, you will not be asked a question that requires typing a word, short answer, or abbreviation.

To answer these types of questions, several test-taking strategies are important. The first strategy is to always follow the directions on the computer screen. Next, use the erasable noteboard that you are provided to set up the formula and the problem to be solved and then perform the calculation. Finally, verify your answer using the on-screen calculator. This will ensure that you have calculated the problem correctly.

In a medication calculation question, the directions may indicate to type in only the numerical component of the answer. In other words, if the answer to a question is 1.4 mL, type only 1.4 if the directions indicate to do so. Additionally, a medication calculation question may ask you to round the answer to the nearest tenth. If so, you must round the answer for it to be correct. For example, if the answer to a medication calculation is 2.33 and you are asked to round to the nearest tenth, then you must type in the answer as 2.3. In a medication calculation question it is also important to remember to place a zero before a decimal point in the answer and to *avoid* placing trailing zeroes in the answer following the decimal point. For example, if the answer is five tenths, type in 0.5 *not* .5 and *not* 0.50 or .50.

In an intravenous flow rate or intravenous infusion time question, the directions may indicate to round the answer to the nearest whole number. If so, then you must type in the answer as a whole number. For example, if the answer is 21.4 drops/min, type the answer as 21.

BOX 1-6 ▲ FILL-IN-THE-BLANK: SAMPLE QUESTION

A client drank 6 oz of juice and 8 oz of tea for breakfast; 4 oz of water to swallow medications at 9 AM and 1 PM; and 8 oz of milk and 8 oz of coffee for lunch. The nurse determines that the client consumed how many milliliters of fluid?

Answer: _____ mL

Answer: 1140

Test-Taking Strategy: This fill-in-the-blank question requires that you calculate the total intake. Read the data in the question carefully and note that the client drank 4 oz of water at both 9 AM and 1 PM. Note that the data in the question are expressed in ounces and you are required to convert ounces to milliliters. Use the erasable noteboard to set up the data and add the total ounces, and verify the amount using the on-screen calculator. Convert the total number of ounces to milliliters, recalling that there are 30 mL in 1 oz. Therefore 6 oz of juice, 8 oz of tea, 4 oz of water at 9 AM, 4 oz of water at 1 PM, 8 oz of milk, and 8 oz of coffee total 38 oz. To convert to milliliters, multiply 38 by 30 to yield 1140 mL.

References
Harkreader H, Hogan MA: *Fundamentals of nursing: caring and clinical judgment*, ed 2, Philadelphia, 2004, Saunders, p 575.
Kee J, Marshall S: *Clinical calculations: with applications to general and specialty areas*, ed 5, Philadelphia, 2004, Saunders, p 28.

In an intake and output calculation question, be certain to read the data carefully. These types of questions may require that you convert ounces to milliliters. If you read the data carefully, you will note specifically what the question requires and will answer correctly. Box 1-5 summarizes these test-taking strategies, and Box 1-6 provides a sample fill-in-the-blank question.

WHAT TEST-TAKING STRATEGIES ARE HELPFUL FOR ANSWERING MULTIPLE-RESPONSE QUESTIONS?

In a multiple-response question, you will be asked to select or check all the correct options that pertain to the question. These questions require you to use the computer mouse and click in a small box next to the options you select. Multiple-response questions can ask about various nursing content areas, such as nursing interventions, expected assessment findings, intended medication effects, medication side effects or adverse effects, or expected responses to treatment. You need to do exactly as the question asks and select or check *all* the options that apply. There is no partial credit given for correct selections. Remember, all correct options must be selected for the answer to be correct. If all the correct options are not selected or if you select all the correct options plus an incorrect option, then the answer to the question will be incorrect.

When answering these types of questions, some test-taking strategies can be of assistance. Always read

BOX 1-7 ▲ POSITIVE AND NEGATIVE EVENT QUERIES

Positive Event Query: Uses strategic words that ask you to select an option that is correct; for example, the event query may read: Which statement by the client *indicates an understanding* of the side effects of the prescribed medication?

Negative Event Query: Uses strategic words that ask you to select an option that is an incorrect item or statement; for example, the event query may read: Which statement by the client *indicates a need for further teaching* about the side effects of the prescribed medication?

the data carefully in the question and determine exactly what the question is asking, or the subject of the question. Look for strategic words (words that focus your attention on critical points when answering the question) and then determine whether the question identifies a positive or a negative event query. (Box 1-7) For example, the side effects of a medication are different from adverse effects, so focusing on the subject of the question is critical. Once you have determined the subject of the question, use nursing knowledge and clinical learning experiences to assist in determining the correct answers. If a disorder is presented in the question, think about the disorder and its associated pathophysiology. Another helpful strategy to use when answering a multiple-response question is to visualize the situation in the question and think about what applies to the situation. In other words, form a mental image of the situation. Box 1-8 summarizes these test-taking strategies, and Box 1-9 provides a sample multiple-response question.

WHAT TEST-TAKING STRATEGIES ARE HELPFUL FOR ANSWERING PRIORITIZING (ORDERED RESPONSE/DRAG AND DROP) QUESTIONS?

In a prioritizing (ordered response) question, you may be asked to use the computer mouse to "drag and drop" the answers presented in order of priority. These questions usually ask you to prioritize nursing interventions or steps in a procedure. Information is presented in a question and, based on the data, you need to determine what you will do first, second, third, and

so forth. You can use three helpful test-taking strategies to answer prioritizing questions: the ABCs (airway, breathing, and circulation), Maslow's hierarchy of needs theory, and the steps of the nursing process.

The ABCs

The ABCs indicate airway, breathing, and circulation and direct the order of priority of nursing actions. Airway is always the first priority in caring for any client. When you are presented with a prioritizing (ordered response) question, use the ABCs to assist in determining the correct order of action. If an option addresses A (airway), that will be your first action. If none of the options addresses airway, then move to B (breathing), followed by C (circulation).

Maslow's Hierarchy of Needs Theory

Abraham Maslow theorized that human needs are satisfied in a particular order, and he arranged human needs in a pyramid or hierarchy (Figure 1-1). According to Maslow, basic physiologic needs such as airway, breathing, circulation, water, food, and elimination are the priority. These basic physiologic needs are followed by safety, and then the psychosocial needs, including security, love and belonging, self-esteem, and self-actualization, in that order. Maslow's hierarchy of needs theory is a helpful guide to prioritize client needs. When you answer prioritizing (ordered response) questions, physiologic needs are the priority and require your immediate attention. Safety needs are the next priority, followed by psychosocial needs.

The Steps of the Nursing Process

The nursing process provides a systematic method for providing care to a client. These steps include

BOX 1-8 ▲ TEST-TAKING STRATEGIES: MULTIPLE RESPONSE

- Always read the data carefully in the question.
- Determine exactly what the question is asking (subject of the question).
- Identify strategic words.
- Note whether the question contains a positive or a negative event query.
- Use nursing knowledge and clinical learning experiences.
- Think about the pathophysiology associated with the disorder, if a disorder is presented in the question.
- Visualize the situation in the question and think about what applies.
- Form a mental image of the situation.

BOX 1-9 ▲ MULTIPLE RESPONSE: SAMPLE QUESTION

A nurse is caring for a client receiving intravenous (IV) therapy who is exhibiting manifestations of circulatory overload. What nursing interventions should the nurse take? Select all that apply.

- ❑ 1 Remove the IV.
- ❑ 2 Monitor vital signs.
- ❑ 3 Notify the physician.
- ❑ 4 Prepare to administer oxygen.
- ❑ 5 Place the client in an upright position.
- ❑ 6 Prepare to administer an antidiuretic hormone.

Answer: 2, 3, 4, 5

Test-Taking Strategy: This multiple-response question requires that you select *all* interventions in the care of a client with circulatory overload, which is the subject of the question. Think about the pathophysiology associated with circulatory overload and recall that it results from excess fluid in the circulatory system; this will assist in determining that a diuretic will be prescribed (not an antidiuretic hormone). Visualizing the situation and forming a mental image of the situation will assist in determining that removing the IV is an incorrect action because an IV access is needed to administer emergency medications.

Reference
Ignatavicius D, Workman M: *Medical surgical nursing: critical thinking for collaborative care,* ed 5, Philadelphia, 2006, Saunders, p 262.

assessment, analysis, planning, implementation, and evaluation (Figure 1-2). These steps are usually followed in sequence, with assessment being the first step and evaluation being the last. Once the nursing process begins, it becomes a cyclical process. The steps of the nursing process can be used as a guide to help you to answer prioritizing (ordered response) questions. The only exception to the rule of selecting an assessment action as the first action is if the situation in the question presents a life-threatening emergency. In such questions, read carefully; an intervention may be the first action.

Additional Helpful Test-Taking Strategies

In addition to the ABCs, Maslow's hierarchy of needs theory, and the steps of the nursing process, some additional helpful pyramid points and strategies will assist in determining the correct order of action (Box 1-10). Box 1-11 provides a sample prioritizing (ordered response) question.

WHAT TEST-TAKING STRATEGIES ARE HELPFUL FOR ANSWERING FIGURE/ ILLUSTRATION QUESTIONS?

In a figure/illustration question you are provided with a visual item and need to answer the question based on that item. Some examples of figures or illustrations that you may note on the examination include rhythm strips, orthopedic or other assistive client devices, anatomic areas of the body, or medication labels. Some figure/illustration questions are in a multiple-choice format. In other words, you are presented with a visual item and a question and, based on this information, you need to answer by selecting one of the four presented options. Other figure/illustration questions may be in the fill-in-the-blank format and require that you type in an answer. For example, you are provided with a medication label and a question that requires a medication calculation and typing in the answer. The important concept to remember is that a figure/illustration question could be presented

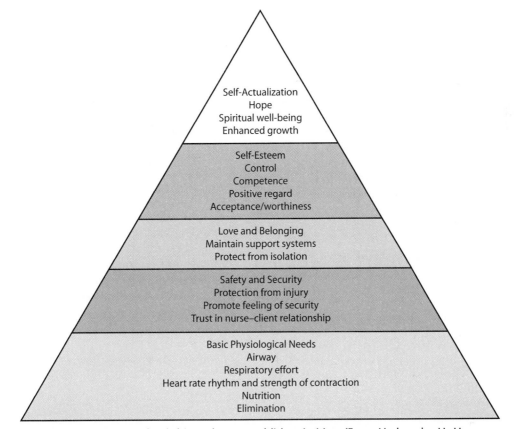

FIGURE 1-1 Using Maslow's hierarchy to establish priorities. (From Harkreader H, Hogan MA: *Fundamentals of nursing: caring and clinical judgment,* ed 2, Philadelphia, 2004, Saunders.)

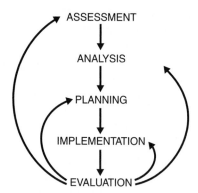

ASSESSMENT

ANALYSIS

PLANNING

IMPLEMENTATION

EVALUATION

FIGURE 1-2 The nursing process cycle. (From Ignatavicius D, Workman M: *Medical surgical nursing: critical thinking for collaborative care,* ed 5, Philadelphia, 2006, Saunders.)

in any format, including multiple choice, fill-in-the-blank, multiple response, prioritizing (ordered response), or chart/exhibit.

Several strategies are helpful when answering figure/illustration questions. The first strategy is to read all the data in the question carefully and focus on the figure/illustration. Think about what the figure/illustration represents, and ask yourself, "What is the question asking?" This strategy will assist you in focusing on the subject of the question. Once you have determined the subject of the question, look for strategic words and use nursing knowledge and clinical learning experiences to answer correctly. If the question is in the fill-in-the-blank format, be certain

BOX 1-10 ▲ TEST-TAKING STRATEGIES: PRIORITIZING (ORDERED RESPONSE/DRAG AND DROP)

Use the ABCs: airway, breathing, and circulation.

Use Maslow's hierarchy of needs theory.

Use the steps of the nursing process.

Look for strategic words.

Determine whether the question identifies a positive or negative event query.

Visualize or form a mental image of the client or clinical event.

Use teaching and learning principles.

Remember that:

- Hands are always washed before any client contact.

- Treatments and procedures are always explained to the client before implementation.

- The nurse checks for a signed informed consent before any invasive procedure.

- Documenting a client's condition and response to treatment is done after care and implementation of treatments.

BOX 1-11 ▲ PRIORITIZING (ORDERED RESPONSE/DRAG AND DROP): SAMPLE QUESTION

The nurse is teaching a client how to use a metered-dose inhaler. In order of priority, list the steps and instructions that the nurse should take to teach the client. (Number 1 is the first step and number 6 is the last step.)

____ Insert the medication canister into the plastic holder.

____ Determine what the client knows about this type of device.

____ Shake the inhaler and remove the cap from the mouthpiece.

____ Hold the breath for a few seconds, remove the mouthpiece, and exhale slowly.

____ Keep the lips secure around the mouthpiece and inhale and push the top of the canister once.

____ Breathe out through the mouth, then place the mouthpiece into the mouth, holding the inhaler upright.

Answer: 2, 1, 3, 6, 5, 4

Test-Taking Strategy: This prioritizing (ordered response) question requires you to list in order of priority the actions that you should take in teaching a client how to use a metered-dose inhaler. Two strategies are important to consider when answering this question. First, use teaching and learning principles, recalling that it is important to first determine what the client knows about this medication administration system. Second, visualize the procedure or form a mental image in your mind as to how this medication system would be used; this strategy will direct you to the correct order for its use.

Reference
Kee J, Marshall S: *Clinical calculations: with applications to general and specialty areas,* ed 5, Philadelphia, 2004, Saunders, pp 69-70.

BOX 1-12 ▲ TEST-TAKING STRATEGIES: FIGURE/ILLUSTRATION

- Read all the data in the question carefully and focus on the figure or illustration.
- Think about what the figure or illustration represents.
- Ask yourself, "What is the question asking?"
- Focus on the subject of the question.
- Look for strategic words.
- Determine whether the question identifies a positive or a negative event query.
- Use nursing knowledge and clinical learning experiences.
- Focus on the question format (fill-in-the-blank, multiple response, prioritizing [ordered response/drag and drop], chart/exhibit), and use the test-taking strategies for answering that type of question.

to use the test-taking strategies for these types of questions and use the erasable noteboard to perform the calculation, verifying the answer with the on-screen calculator. If the question is in the multiple-response, prioritizing (ordered response), or chart/exhibit format, use the test-taking strategies for answering these types of questions and remember to visualize the situation in the question and form a mental image of the situation. The test-taking strategies for figure/illustration questions are listed in Box 1-12. Box 1-13 provides a sample figure/illustration question.

WHAT TEST-TAKING STRATEGIES ARE HELPFUL FOR ANSWERING CHART/EXHIBIT QUESTIONS?

A chart/exhibit question will most likely provide you with data from a client's medical record and ask you a question about those data. These types of questions may also provide an exhibit of some type, such as a physician's order form with written orders or a laboratory result form listing results from various laboratory tests. These questions will most likely be in the multiple-choice format but may also be presented in other types of alternate item question formats.

Some of the test-taking strategies to answer this type of question are similar to those that you can use for the figure/illustration questions. First, it is critically important to read all the data in the chart or exhibit. Remember, the data are presented to you for a reason, so avoid "skimming over" the information presented. Next, focus on the subject of the question, look for strategic words, and determine whether the question identifies a positive or a negative event query. Once you have determined the subject of the

question, reread the data provided, use nursing knowledge and clinical learning experiences, and identify a relationship between the subject of the question and the data provided. Finally, it is important to note the question format being used (multiple choice, fill-in-the-blank, multiple response, prioritizing [ordered response], figure/illustration) and use the specific test-taking strategies for these question types. These helpful test-taking strategies are listed in Box 1-14. Box 1-15 provides a sample figure/illustration question.

WHAT ARE THE ACCOMPANYING PRODUCTS IN *SAUNDERS PYRAMID TO SUCCESS* FOR THE NCLEX-RN® EXAMINATION?

Several accompanying products will be extremely helpful during your nursing program as you prepare for nursing examinations. At the same time, these products will also prepare you for the NCLEX-RN examination. These accompanying products contain both multiple-choice questions and alternate item format questions. A brief description of each product is described below.

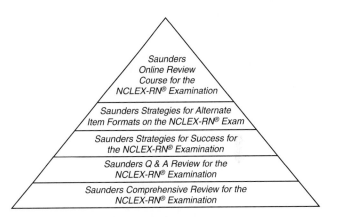

Saunders Comprehensive Review for the NCLEX-RN® Examination

This is an excellent resource to use both while you are in nursing school and in preparation for the NCLEX-RN examination. This book includes both nursing content review and practice questions. It contains 20 units and 76 chapters, each designed to identify specific components of nursing content. The book and accompanying software contain more than 4000 practice questions, both multiple-choice and alternate item format questions.

Saunders Q & A Review for the NCLEX-RN® Examination

This book and accompanying software provide more than 5000 practice questions. The chapters in this

BOX 1-13 ▲ FIGURE/ILLUSTRATION: SAMPLE QUESTION

Biaxin (clarithromycin) granules oral suspension 250 mg twice daily has been prescribed for a client with pharyngitis. How many milliliters should the nurse prepare to administer one dose?

Answer: _____ mL

Answer: 10

Test-Taking Strategy: This figure/illustration question is in a fill-in-the-blank format. In other words, you are required to focus on the figure/illustration of the medication label, perform a calculation to determine the number of milliliters to administer in one dose, and type in the answer. Use nursing knowledge of the formula for medication calculation doses. Perform the calculation on the erasable noteboard, and verify the amount using the on-screen calculator. The formula and calculation are presented below.

Formula

$$\frac{\text{Desired}}{\text{Available}} \times \text{mL} = \text{mL per dose}$$

$$\frac{250 \text{ mg}}{125 \text{ mg}} \times 5 \text{ mL} = 10 \text{ mL}$$

References

Kee J, Marshall S: *Clinical calculations: with applications to general and specialty areas,* ed 5, Philadelphia, 2004, Saunders, p 89.
Mosby's 2006 drug consult for nurses, St Louis, 2006, Mosby, p 167.

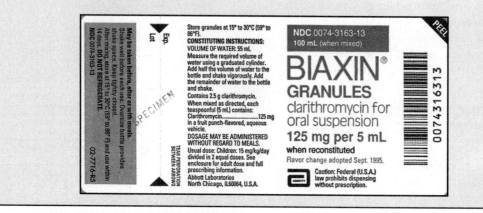

Figure from Kee J, Marshall S: *Clinical calculations: with applications to general and specialty areas,* ed 5, Philadelphia, 2004, Saunders.

BOX 1-14 ▲ TEST-TAKING STRATEGIES: CHART/EXHIBIT

- Read all the data in the chart or exhibit.
- Avoid "skimming over" the information presented.
- Focus on the subject of the question.
- Look for strategic words.
- Determine whether the question identifies a positive or negative event query.

- Reread the data provided and use nursing knowledge and clinical learning experiences to answer correctly.
- Identify a relationship between the subject of the question and the data provided.
- Note the question format being presented, and use the specific test-taking strategies for that type of question.

BOX 1-15 ▲ CHART/EXHIBIT: SAMPLE QUESTION

Prednisone (Deltasone) is prescribed for a hospitalized client with severe rheumatoid arthritis. Which daily laboratory result should the nurse monitor most closely?

❑ 1 Lipase level
❑ 2 Chloride level
❑ 3 Uric acid level
❑ 4 Blood glucose level

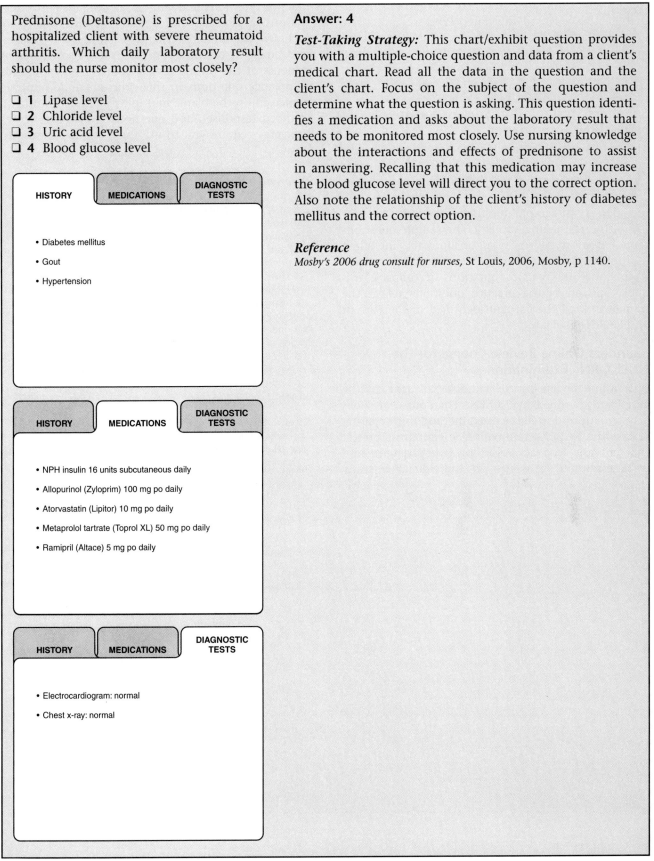

HISTORY | MEDICATIONS | DIAGNOSTIC TESTS

• Diabetes mellitus

• Gout

• Hypertension

HISTORY | **MEDICATIONS** | DIAGNOSTIC TESTS

• NPH insulin 16 units subcutaneous daily

• Allopurinol (Zyloprim) 100 mg po daily

• Atorvastatin (Lipitor) 10 mg po daily

• Metaprolol tartrate (Toprol XL) 50 mg po daily

• Ramipril (Altace) 5 mg po daily

HISTORY | MEDICATIONS | **DIAGNOSTIC TESTS**

• Electrocardiogram: normal

• Chest x-ray: normal

Answer: 4

Test-Taking Strategy: This chart/exhibit question provides you with a multiple-choice question and data from a client's medical chart. Read all the data in the question and the client's chart. Focus on the subject of the question and determine what the question is asking. This question identifies a medication and asks about the laboratory result that needs to be monitored most closely. Use nursing knowledge about the interactions and effects of prednisone to assist in answering. Recalling that this medication may increase the blood glucose level will direct you to the correct option. Also note the relationship of the client's history of diabetes mellitus and the correct option.

Reference
Mosby's 2006 drug consult for nurses, St Louis, 2006, Mosby, p 1140.

book are uniquely designed and are based on the NCLEX-RN examination Test Plan framework, including Client Needs and Integrated Processes. Alternate item format questions are included. With practice questions uniquely focused on the Client Needs and the Integrated Processes, you can assess your level of competence in each area of the Test Plan.

Saunders Strategies for Success for the NCLEX-RN® Examination

This book and accompanying CD provide all the test-taking strategies that will help you pass your nursing examinations and the NCLEX-RN examination. The chapters describe all the test-taking strategies and include several sample questions that illustrate how to use the test-taking strategy. The sample questions represent all types of question formats, including multiple-choice and alternate item format questions. A total of 500 practice questions accompany this book, and all of the practice questions reflect the framework and the content identified in the current NCLEX-RN Test Plan.

Saunders Online Review Course for the NCLEX-RN® Examination

The online review course addresses all areas of the Test Plan identified by NCSBN. The course provides a systematic and individualized method for preparing to take the NCLEX examination. It contains a pretest that provides feedback regarding your strengths and weaknesses and generates an individualized study schedule in a calendar format. Content review with practice questions and case studies, figures and illustrations, a glossary, and animations and videos are included. A cumulative examination and a computerized adaptive examination (CAT) are also key components of the online review course. The thousands of practice questions in this course include multiple choice, fill-in-the-blank, multiple response, prioritizing (ordered response), and questions containing figures that may require you to use the computer mouse to answer.

References

Chernecky C, Berger B: *Laboratory tests and diagnostic procedures,* ed 4, Philadelphia, 2004, Saunders.

Harkreader H, Hogan MA: *Fundamentals of nursing: caring and clinical judgment,* ed 2, Philadelphia, 2004, Saunders.

Ignatavicius D, Workman M: *Medical surgical nursing: critical thinking for collaborative care,* ed 5, Philadelphia, 2006, Saunders.

Kee J, Marshall S: *Clinical calculations: with applications to general and specialty areas,* ed 5, Philadelphia, 2004, Saunders.

Mosby's 2006 drug consult for nurses, St Louis, 2005, Mosby.

National Council of State Boards of Nursing: www.ncsbn.org.

National Council of State Boards of Nursing: *National Council of State Boards of Nursing Test Plan for the NCLEX-RN® Examination* (effective date: April 2007), Chicago, 2006, The Council.

Silvestri L: *Saunders Q & A review for the NCLEX-RN® examination,* ed 3, Philadelphia, 2006, Saunders.

Silvestri L: *Saunders comprehensive review for the NCLEX-RN® examination,* ed 3, Philadelphia, 2005, Saunders.

Silvestri L: *Saunders strategies for success for the NCLEX-RN® examination,* ed 3, Philadelphia, 2005, Saunders.

CHAPTER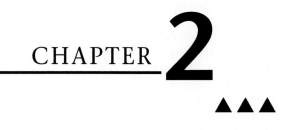

Safe and Effective Care Environment Questions

The Safe and Effective Care Environment category of Client Needs includes two subcategories: Management of Care and Safety and Infection Control. According to the National Council of State Boards of Nursing (NCSBN), Management of Care makes up 13% to 19% of the questions on the examination, and Safety and Infection Control makes up 8% to 14% of the questions (Box 2-1). Following is a description of each subcategory and its associated content. Refer to the *National Council of State Boards of Nursing Test Plan for the NCLEX-RN® Examination* (2006) on the NCSBN website at www.ncsbn.org for additional information. Practice questions that address content in each subcategory follows the descriptions.

Management of Care

According to the NCSBN, Management of Care (13% to 19%) questions test the nurse's knowledge, skill, and ability to provide and direct nursing care that will enhance the care delivery setting to protect clients, families, significant others, visitors, and health care personnel. Some of the content related to this subcategory is identified in Box 2-2.

Safety and Infection Control

According to the NCSBN, Safety and Infection Control (8% to 14%) questions test the nurse's role and responsibilities required to protect clients, families, significant others, visitors, and health care personnel from health and environmental hazards. Some of the content related to this subcategory is identified in Box 2-3.

BOX 2-1 ▲ SAFE AND EFFECTIVE CARE ENVIRONMENT

Management of Care = 13% to 19% of the questions

Safety and Infection Control = 8% to 14% of the questions

BOX 2-2 ▲ MANAGEMENT OF CARE CONTENT

- Acting as a client advocate
- Applying management concepts in the care of clients
- Collaborating and consulting with other health care team members
- Delegating care and supervising other health care team members
- Educating other health care team members
- Ensuring client's decisions are incorporated in advance directives
- Ensuring client rights are upheld, including confidentiality and informed consent
- Establishing priorities of care
- Identifying appropriate referrals for clients
- Identifying ethical and legal issues related to client care
- Managing resources, including supplies and equipment, cost-effectively
- Participating in performance improvement (quality improvement) programs
- Providing care based on case management concepts
- Providing continuity of care
- Using information technology systems and maintaining information security measures

BOX 2-3 ▲ SAFETY AND INFECTION CONTROL CONTENT

- Employing methods of medical and surgical asepsis
- Handling hazardous and infectious material
- Identifying the nurse's role in disaster planning and preparing and implementing an emergency response plan
- Implementing standard, transmission-based, and other precautions
- Participating in security plan activities, including triage and evacuation procedures
- Preventing accidents and errors
- Preventing injuries and ensuring home safety
- Reporting accidents or errors and documenting on incident or other reports
- Using ergonomic principles in the workplace
- Using restraints, safety devices, and equipment safely

PRACTICE QUESTIONS

Chart/Exhibit with a Prioritizing (Ordered Response)

1. A hospital-based home care nurse works a 12-hour day shift (7 AM to 7 PM) and is planning client home visits/activities for the day and has the following list of visits/activities noted on a worksheet to carry out. The hospital laboratory and the clients' home addresses are within a 5-mile radius. List in order of priority how the nurse would best plan the client visits/activities. (Number 1 is the first visit/activity and number 6 is the last visit/activity.)

CHART/EXHIBIT
WORKSHEET: VISITS/ACTIVITIES

____ Obtain a fasting blood glucose specimen from a client who has diabetes mellitus and takes NPH insulin daily in the morning.

____ Administer the first dose of eye drops to a client with glaucoma who requires twice daily administration.

____ Perform the first dressing change on a client with a foot ulcer who requires twice daily dressing changes.

____ Perform the second dressing change on a client with a foot ulcer who requires twice daily dressing changes.

____ Administer the second dose of eye drops to a client with glaucoma who requires twice daily administration.

____ Conduct a home care admission assessment on a client who was discharged from the hospital with a diagnosis of resolved pneumonia.

Answer: 1, 2, 3, 6, 5, 4

Rationale: When planning the order of priority for care, the nurse should consider several factors. Primarily the nurse needs to consider the clients' needs and the time that it may take to perform each task or activity. In this situation, the nurse should first obtain the fasting blood glucose specimen from a client who has diabetes mellitus and takes NPH insulin daily in the morning because the client is unable to take the insulin or consume food until this is done. The nurse would next plan to visit the client to administer the first dose of eye drops and then visit the client with a foot ulcer to change the dressing, since both clients require twice daily treatments and it is best to schedule these treatments as far apart as possible. Since administering eye drops would take less time than a dressing change, the nurse would visit the client requiring the eye drops before the client requiring the dressing change. Since an admission assessment takes time the nurse would perform this next. Also, there are no data that indicate the client with resolving pneumonia requiring admission has immediate needs. Finally, the nurse should revisit the clients requiring the second administration of eye drops and a dressing change, in that order.

Test-Taking Strategy: To answer this question, use the principles related to prioritizing and time management. Read each activity and consider both the clients' needs and the time that it may take to perform the activity. This will assist in identifying the best order of action. Review the guidelines related to prioritizing and time management if you had difficulty with this question.

Level of Cognitive Ability: Application
Client Needs: Safe and Effective Care Environment
Integrated Process: Nursing Process/Planning
Content Area: Management of Care

References
Harkreader H, Hogan MA: *Fundamentals of nursing: caring and clinical judgment,* ed 2, Philadelphia, 2004, Saunders, p 281.
Potter P, Perry A: *Fundamentals of nursing,* ed 6, St Louis, 2005, Mosby, pp 318-320, 378.

Prioritizing (Ordered Response)

2. List in order of priority the steps involved in processing an ethical dilemma. (Number 1 is the first step and number 6 is the last step.)

   ___ Evaluate the action.
   ___ Negotiate the outcome.
   ___ Consider possible courses of action.
   ___ Verbalize the problem or ethical dilemma.
   ___ Examine and determine own values on the ethical issue.
   ___ Gather information relevant to the clinical situation and determine if a true ethical dilemma exists.

Answer: 6, 5, 4, 3, 2, 1

Rationale: An ethical dilemma exists when a problem arises that causes distress, confusion, or conflict for clients and caregivers. Processing an ethical dilemma requires negotiation of differences, incorporation of conflicting ideas, and an effort to respect differences of opinions. The first step in processing an ethical dilemma is to gather all the information relevant to the situation to ensure that a true dilemma exists, since occasionally an overlooked fact may provide quick resolution. Once this has been determined, the nurse should examine and identify his or her own values on the ethical issue (second step). This is known as values clarification and provides the foundation for clarity during necessary discussions when resolving the dilemma. Step 3 involves verbalizing the problem. Agreeing to the statement of the problem will help those involved to proceed toward resolution in a focused manner. Once the problem is clearly identified, all possible courses of action can be considered. Considering all possible courses of action will reflect opinions that conflict (step 4). Step 5 involves negotiation of the outcome based on all possible courses of action and points of view. In the best of circumstances, all involved will discover a course of action that is acceptable to everyone. Finally, as the last step, the action is evaluated to ensure the course of action taken is acceptable.

Test-Taking Strategy: Focus on the subject, the steps in processing an ethical dilemma. Use the steps of the nursing process; recalling the systematic order of these steps—assessment, analysis, planning, implementation, and evaluation—will assist in answering this question. Review the steps in processing an ethical dilemma if you had difficulty with this question.

Level of Cognitive Ability: Application
Client Needs: Safe and Effective Care Environment
Integrated Process: Nursing Process/Implementation
Content Area: Management of Care

Reference
Potter P, Perry A: *Fundamentals of nursing*, ed 6, St Louis, 2005, Mosby, pp 398-399.

Multiple Response

3. A nurse caring for a client with end-stage renal failure is asked by a family member about advance directives. Which statements should the nurse include when discussing advance directives with the client's family member? Select all that apply.

   ❑ **1** Two witnesses, either a relative or physician, are needed when the client signs a living will.

   ❑ **2** The determination of decisional capacity of a client is usually made by the physician and family.

   ❑ **3** A health care proxy can write a living will for a client if the client becomes incompetent and unable to do so.

   ❑ **4** Living wills are written documents that direct treatment in accordance with a client's wishes in the event of a terminal illness or condition.

   ❑ **5** Under the Patient Self-Determination Act (PSDA) (1991), it must be documented in the client's record whether the client has signed an advance directive.

   ❑ **6** For advance directives to be enforceable, the client must be legally incompetent or lack decisional capacity to make decisions regarding health care treatment.

Answer: 2, 4, 5, 6

Rationale: The two basic advance directives are living wills and durable powers of attorney for health care. Under the PSDA, it must be documented in the client's record whether the client has signed an advance directive. For living wills or durable powers of attorney for health care to be enforceable, the client must be legally incompetent or lack decisional capacity to make decisions regarding health care treatment. The determination of decisional capacity is usually made by the physician and family, whereas the determination of legal competency is made by a judge. Living wills are written documents that direct treatment in accordance with a client's wishes in the event of a terminal illness or condition. Generally, two witnesses, neither of whom can be a relative or physician, are needed when the client signs the document. A durable power of attorney for health care designates an agent, surrogate, or proxy to make health care decisions if and when the client is no longer able to make decisions on his or her own behalf; however, a health care proxy cannot legally write a living will for a client.

Test-Taking Strategy: Focus on the subject, the characteristics of advance directives. Read each option carefully. Recalling that these are legal documents based on the client's wishes will assist in determining the correct options. Review the characteristics of advance directives if you had difficulty with this question.

Level of Cognitive Ability: Application
Client Needs: Safe and Effective Care Environment
Integrated Process: Nursing Process/Implementation
Content Area: Management of Care

Reference
Potter P, Perry A: *Fundamentals of nursing*, ed 6, St Louis, 2005, Mosby, pp 408-410.

Multiple Response

4. A nurse is developing an educational session on client advocacy for the nursing staff. The nurse plans to tell the nursing staff that which of the following are examples of the nurse acting as a client advocate? Select all that apply.

   ❏ 1 Obtaining an informed consent for a surgical procedure
   ❏ 2 Providing information necessary for a client to make informed decisions
   ❏ 3 Telling a client that he or she will need to defend himself or herself about health care rights
   ❏ 4 Providing assistance in asserting the client's human and legal rights if the need arises
   ❏ 5 Ignoring the client's religious or cultural beliefs when assisting the client in making an informed decision
   ❏ 6 Defending the client's rights by speaking out against policies or actions that might endanger the client's well-being

Answer: 2, 4, 6

Rationale: In the role of client advocate, the nurse protects the client's human and legal rights and provides assistance in asserting those rights if the need arises. The nurse advocates for the client, keeping in mind the client's religion and culture. The nurse also defends clients' rights in a general way by speaking out against policies or actions that might endanger the client's well-being or conflict with his or her rights. Informed consent is part of the physician-client relationship; in most situations, obtaining clients' informed consent does not fall within the nursing duty. Even though the nurse assumes the responsibility for witnessing the client's signature on the consent form, the nurse does not legally assume the duty of obtaining informed consent.

Test-Taking Strategy: Focus on the subject, examples of the nurse acting as a client advocate, and read each option carefully. Focus on the definition of a client advocate. Remembering that in this role the nurse protects the client's human and legal rights and provides assistance in asserting those rights if the need arises will assist in selecting the correct examples. Review the nurse's role as a client advocate if you had difficulty with this question.

Level of Cognitive Ability: Application
Client Needs: Safe and Effective Care Environment
Integrated Process: Caring
Content Area: Management of Care

Reference
Potter P, Perry A: *Fundamentals of nursing,* ed 6, St Louis, 2005, pp 19, 416.

Multiple Response

5. Which of the following are characteristics of case management? Select all that apply.

   ❑ 1 A case manager usually does not provide direct care.
   ❑ 2 Critical pathways and CareMaps are types of case management.
   ❑ 3 A case manager does not need to be concerned with standards of cost management.
   ❑ 4 A case manager collaborates with and supervises the care delivered by other staff members.
   ❑ 5 A case manager coordinates a hospitalized client's acute care and follows up with the client after discharge to home.
   ❑ 6 The evaluation process involves continuous monitoring and analysis of the needs of the client and services provided.

Answer: 1, 4, 5, 6

Rationale: Case management is a care management approach that coordinates heath care services to clients and their families while maintaining quality of care and minimizing health care costs. Case managers usually do not provide direct care; instead they collaborate with and supervise the care delivered by other staff members and actively coordinate client discharge planning. A case manager is usually held accountable for some standard of cost management. A case manager coordinates a hospitalized client's acute care, follows up with the client after discharge to home, and is responsible and accountable for appraising the overall usefulness and effectiveness of the case managed services. This evaluation process involves continuous monitoring and analysis of the client's needs and services provided. Critical pathways or CareMaps are not types of case management; rather, they are multidisciplinary treatment plans used in a case management delivery system to implement timely interventions in a coordinated care plan.

Test-Taking Strategy: Focus on the subject, the characteristics of case management, and read each option carefully. Recall that case management is a care management approach that coordinates heath care services to clients and their families while maintaining quality of care and keeping health care costs at a minimum. This will assist in selecting the correct options. Review the characteristics of case management if you had difficulty with this question.

Level of Cognitive Ability: Comprehension
Client Needs: Safe and Effective Care Environment
Integrated Process: Nursing Process/Planning
Content Area: Management of Care

References

Cohen E, Cesta T: *Nursing case management: from essentials to advanced practice applications,* ed 4, St Louis, 2005, Mosby, pp 22-23.
Potter P, Perry A: *Fundamentals of nursing,* ed 6, St Louis, 2005, p 373.

Multiple Response

6. A nurse manager is developing an educational session for nursing staff on the components of informed consent and the information to be shared with a client to obtain informed consent. Select the information that the nurse manager should include in the session. Select all that apply.

   ❑ 1 The nurse is responsible for providing information about tests, procedures, and treatments, including the complications and risks involved.
   ❑ 2 The client needs to be informed of the prognosis if the test, procedure, or treatment is refused.
   ❑ 3 The client cannot refuse a test, procedure, or treatment once the test, procedure, or treatment is started.
   ❑ 4 The name(s) of the persons performing the test or procedure or providing treatment should be documented on the informed consent form.
   ❑ 5 A description of the complications and risks of the test, procedure, or treatment, as well as anticipated pain or discomfort, needs to be explained to the client.
   ❑ 6 The nurse is responsible for obtaining the client's signature on an informed consent form even if the client has questions about the test, procedure, or treatment to be performed.

Answer: 2, 4, 5

Rationale: Informed consent is a person's agreement to allow something to happen based on full disclosure of risks, benefits, alternatives, and consequences of refusal. The physician is responsible for conveying information and obtaining the informed consent. The nurse may be the person who actually ensures that the client signs the informed consent form; however, the nurse does this only after the physician has instructed the client and it has been determined that the client has understood the information. The following factors are required for informed consent: a brief, complete explanation of the test, procedure, or treatment; names and qualifications of persons performing and assisting in the test, procedure, or treatment; a description of the complications and risks as well as anticipated pain or discomfort; an explanation of alternative therapies to the proposed test, procedure, or treatment as well as the risks of doing nothing; and his or her right to refuse the test, procedure, or treatment even after it has been started.

Test-Taking Strategy: To answer this question correctly, there are two primary factors to bear in mind. The first factor is that the physician is responsible for conveying information and obtaining the informed consent. The second factor is that the client has the right to be fully informed. Bearing these factors in mind will assist in answering this question and other questions related to informed consent. Review the issues surrounding informed consent if you had difficulty with this question.

Level of Cognitive Ability: Application
Client Needs: Safe and Effective Care Environment
Integrated Process: Nursing Process/Planning
Content Area: Management of Care

References
Harkreader H, Hogan MA: *Fundamentals of nursing: caring and clinical judgment,* ed 2, Philadelphia, 2004, Saunders, p 36.
Potter P, Perry A: *Fundamentals of nursing,* ed 6, St Louis, 2005, Mosby, pp 82, 416.

Multiple Response

7. A nurse is planning client and unit activities for the day. Select the activities that the nurse should delegate to the nursing assistant. Select all that apply.

    ❑ **1** Deliver fresh water to clients.
    ❑ **2** Empty urine out of Foley bags.
    ❑ **3** Take temperatures, pulses, respirations, and blood pressures.
    ❑ **4** Count the substance control medications in the narcotic medication supply.
    ❑ **5** Check the crash cart (cardiopulmonary resuscitation cart) for necessary supplies using a checklist.
    ❑ **6** Check all intravenous (IV) solution bags on clients receiving IV therapy for the remaining amounts of solution in the bags.

Answer: 1, 2, 3

Rationale: Delegation is the transfer of responsibility for the performance of an activity or task while retaining account-ability for the outcome. When delegating an activity, the nurse needs to consider the educational preparation and experience of the individual. A nursing assistant is trained to perform noninvasive tasks and tasks that meet basic client needs. The nursing assistant is also trained to take vital signs. Therefore the appropriate activities to assign to the nursing assistant would be to empty urine out of Foley bags; deliver fresh water to clients; and take temperatures, pulses, respirations, and blood pressures. Any activities related to medications and IV therapy need to be delegated to a licensed nurse. Although a nursing assistant is trained in performing cardiopulmonary resuscitation, he or she is not trained to check a crash cart, and this activity needs to be assigned to a licensed nurse.

Test-Taking Strategy: Focus on the subject of the question, activities to be delegated to a nursing assistant. Recalling that a nursing assistant is trained to perform noninvasive tasks and that medication and IV therapy and any activity that re-quires critical thinking skills need to be delegated to a licensed nurse will assist in answering this question. Review the prin-ciples related to delegation of activities if you had difficulty with this question.

Level of Cognitive Ability: Application
Client Needs: Safe and Effective Care Environment
Integrated Process: Nursing Process/Planning
Content Area: Management of Care

Reference
Potter P, Perry A: *Fundamentals of nursing*, ed 6, St Louis, 2005, Mosby, pp 379-380.

Multiple Response

8. A nurse is developing a hospital policy on guidelines for telephone and verbal orders. Which of the following guidelines should the nurse include in the policy? Select all that apply.

   ❏ 1 The nurse should clarify questions with the physician.
   ❏ 2 The nurse should repeat the prescribed orders back to the physician.
   ❏ 3 Verbal orders are never acceptable; the physician must document the order.
   ❏ 4 The use of abbreviations such as TO (telephone order) is never acceptable.
   ❏ 5 Cosigning the order by the physician is not necessary if the nurse repeats the order for verification.
   ❏ 6 The name of the physician giving the order does not need to be documented if the physician giving the order is the client's primary physician.

Answer: 1, 2

Rationale: A telephone order (TO) involves a physician stating a prescribed therapy over the phone to a nurse. Telephone orders are frequently given at night or during an emergency and need to be given only when absolutely necessary. Likewise, a verbal order (VO) is acceptable when there is no opportunity for the physician to write the order such as in an emergency situation. Additional guidelines for telephone and verbal orders include the following: clearly determine the client's name, room number, and diagnosis; repeat any prescribed orders back to the physician; use clarifying questions to avoid misunderstandings; write TO (telephone order) or VO (verbal order), including the date and time, name of the client, complete order, name of the physician giving the order, and nurse taking the order; and have the physician cosign the order within the time frame designated by the health care agency (usually 24 hours).

Test-Taking Strategy: Focus on the subject, guidelines for taking telephone and verbal orders. You can easily eliminate options 3 and 4 because of the close-ended word "never" in these options. Next eliminate option 5 because of the words "not necessary" and option 6 because the order needs to indicate the prescribing physician. Also, reading each option carefully and thinking about the legal issues related to physicians' orders will assist in answering correctly. Review the guidelines for telephone and verbal orders if you had difficulty with this question.

Level of Cognitive Ability: Application
Client Needs: Safe and Effective Care Environment
Integrated Process: Nursing Process/Implementation
Content Area: Management of Care

Reference
Potter P, Perry A: *Fundamentals of nursing*, ed 6, St Louis, 2005, Mosby, p 497.

Multiple Response

9. A nurse is reading the history and physical examination of an older client admitted to the hospital. Which findings documented in the history place the client at risk for accidents? Select all that apply.

   ❑ 1 Range of motion is limited.
   ❑ 2 Peripheral vision is decreased.
   ❑ 3 No client complaints of nocturia.
   ❑ 4 Transmission of hot impulses is delayed.
   ❑ 5 High-frequency hearing tones are perceptible.
   ❑ 6 Voluntary and autonomic reflexes are slowed.

Answer: 1, 2, 4, 6

Rationale: The physiologic changes that occur during the aging process increase the client's risk for accidents. Musculo-skeletal changes include a decrease in muscle strength and function, lessened joint mobility, and limited range of motion. Nervous system changes include slowed voluntary and autonomic reflexes. Sensory changes include a decrease in peripheral vision and lens accommodation, delayed transmission of hot and cold impulses, and impaired hearing as high-frequency tones become less perceptible. Genitourinary changes include nocturia and incontinence.

Test-Taking Strategy: Focus on the subject, the findings that place the older client at risk for accidents. Reading each option carefully and keeping in mind the factors that affect client safety will assist in answering the question. Review the factors that place a client at risk for accidents if you had difficulty with this question.

Level of Cognitive Ability: Comprehension
Client Needs: Safe and Effective Care Environment
Integrated Process: Nursing Process/Assessment
Content Area: Safety and Infection Control

Reference
Potter P, Perry A: *Fundamentals of nursing,* ed 6, St Louis, 2005, Mosby, p 965.

Figure/Illustration with a Multiple Response

10. The nurse plans to wear this protective device (refer to figure) when caring for clients with which of the following disorders? Select all that apply.

❏ 1 Scabies
❏ 2 Tuberculosis
❏ 3 Hepatitis A virus
❏ 4 Pharyngeal diphtheria
❏ 5 Respiratory viral influenza
❏ 6 Meningococcal pneumonia

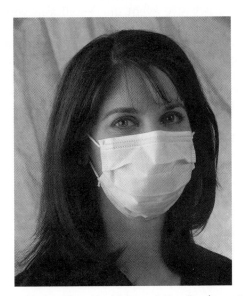

From Harkreader H, Hogan MA: *Fundamentals of nursing: caring and clinical judgment,* ed 2, Philadelphia, 2004, Saunders. Courtesy Medline Industries Inc.

Answer: 4, 5, 6

Rationale: A standard mask is used as part of droplet precautions to protect the nurse from acquiring the client's infection. Droplet precautions refer to precautions used for organisms that can spread through the air but are unable to remain in the air farther than 3 feet. Many respiratory viral infections such as respiratory viral influenza require the use of a standard mask when caring for the client. Some other disorders requiring the use of a standard mask include pharyngeal diphtheria; rubella; streptococcal pharyngitis; pertussis; mumps; pneumonia, including meningococcal pneumonia; and the pneumonic plague. Scabies and hepatitis A are transmitted by direct contact with an infected person and require the use of contact precautions for protection. Tuberculosis requires the use of airborne precautions and the use of an individually fitted particulate filter mask. A standard mask would not protect the nurse from *Mycobacterium tuberculosis.*

Test-Taking Strategy: Focus on the figure and note that it is a standard mask. This indicates the need for the nurse to protect himself or herself from inhaling an organism. You can eliminate option 2 by recalling that tuberculosis requires the use of an individually fitted particulate filter mask. Next eliminate options 1 and 3 by recalling that these infections are not transmitted by the respiratory route. Noting that options 4, 5, and 6 are respiratory disorders will assist in answering correctly. Review the indications for the use of a standard mask if you had difficulty with this question.

Level of Cognitive Ability: Application
Client Needs: Safe and Effective Care Environment
Integrated Process: Nursing Process/Implementation
Content Area: Safety and Infection Control

References

Harkreader H, Hogan MA: *Fundamentals of nursing: caring and clinical judgment,* ed 2, Philadelphia, 2004, Saunders, pp 456, 469-470.
Potter P, Perry A: *Fundamentals of nursing,* ed 6, St Louis, 2005, Mosby, pp 776, 797.

Multiple Response

11. Wrist restraints have been prescribed for a client who is continuously pulling at his gastrostomy tube. The nurse develops a care plan and determines that which of the following are unexpected outcomes related to the use of restraints? Select all that apply.

    ❏ 1 The client is agitated.
    ❏ 2 The client's left hand is pale and cold.
    ❏ 3 The client's skin under the restraint is red.
    ❏ 4 The client verbalizes the reason for the restraints.
    ❏ 5 The client is unable to reach the gastrostomy tube with his hands.
    ❏ 6 The client slips his hand out of the restraint and pulls at his gastrostomy tube.

Answer: 1, 2, 3, 6

Rationale: A physical restraint is a mechanical or physical device used to immobilize a client or extremity. The restraint restricts freedom of movement. Unexpected outcomes in the use of restraints include signs of impaired skin integrity such as redness or skin breakdown; altered neurovascular status such as cyanosis, pallor, coldness of the skin, or complaints of tingling, numbness, or pain; increased confusion, disorientation, or agitation; or escape from the restraint device resulting in a fall or injury. Client verbalization of the reason for the restraints and the client's inability to reach the gastrostomy tube with his hands are expected outcomes.

Test-Taking Strategy: Note the strategic word *unexpected.* This word indicates a negative event query and asks you to select the options that indicate undesirable effects of the use of the restraints. Focusing on the data in the question and recalling the nursing responsibilities related to care of a client in restraints will assist in answering the question. Review the expected and unexpected findings related to the use of restraints if you had difficulty with this question.

Level of Cognitive Ability: Analysis
Client Needs: Safe and Effective Care Environment
Integrated Process: Nursing Process/Evaluation
Content Area: Safety and Infection Control

Reference
Potter P, Perry A: *Fundamentals of nursing,* ed 6, St Louis, 2005, p 989.

Multiple Response

12. A nurse is discussing accident prevention with the family of an older client who is being discharged from the hospital after having hip surgery. Which physical factors place the client at risk for injury at home? Select all that apply.

    ❏ 1 A night-light in the bathroom
    ❏ 2 Elevated toilet seat with armrests
    ❏ 3 Cooking equipment such as a stove
    ❏ 4 Smoke and carbon monoxide detectors
    ❏ 5 A low thermostat setting on the water heater
    ❏ 6 Common household objects such as a doormat

Answer: 3, 6

Rationale: Physical hazards in the environment place the client at risk for accidental injury and death. Adequate lighting such as night-lights in dark hallways and bathrooms reduces the physical hazard by illuminating areas in which a person moves about. An elevated toilet seat with armrests and nonslip strips on the floor in front of the toilet are useful in reducing falls in the bathroom. Cooking equipment and appliances, particularly stoves, can be a main source for in-home fires and fire injuries. Smoke and carbon monoxide detectors should be placed throughout the home to alert members of the household of a potential danger. A low thermostat setting on the water heater reduces the risk of burns during water use such as bathing or showering. Injuries in the home frequently result from tripping over or coming into contact with common household objects such as a doormat, small rugs on the floor or stairs, or clutter around the house.

Test-Taking Strategy: Read each option carefully. Focus on the subject of the question, the physical factors that place the client at risk for injury at home. Next think about whether the factor is safe or presents a potential for injury; this will assist in answering the question. Review the physical factors that place clients at risk for injury if you had difficulty with this question.

Level of Cognitive Ability: Application
Client Needs: Safe and Effective Care Environment
Integrated Process: Teaching and Learning
Content Area: Safety and Infection Control

Reference
Potter P, Perry A: *Fundamentals of nursing*, ed 6, St Louis, 2005, Mosby, p 962.

Figure/Illustration with a Fill-in-the-Blank

13. The nurse should select which anatomic location to safely administer an intramuscular injection in the vastus lateralis muscle of an adult client? (Refer to figure.)

Answer: _____

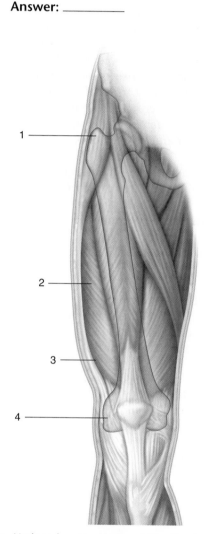

From Harkreader H, Hogan MA: *Fundamentals of nursing: caring and clinical judgment,* ed 2, Philadelphia, 2004, Saunders.

Answer: 2

Rationale: The vastus lateralis muscle is a thick, well-developed muscle located on the anterolateral aspect of the thigh. In the adult, it extends from a handbreadth above the knee to a handbreadth below the greater trochanter. It is best to use this site by injecting the outer middle third of the thigh. There are no large nerves or blood vessels in this area, and the muscle does not lie over a joint. Option 1 identifies the greater trochanter of the femur. Option 3 identifies the lowest area of the vastus lateralis muscle. Option 4 identifies the lateral femoral condyle.

Test-Taking Strategy: Focus on the subject of the question, administration of an intramuscular injection in the vastus lateralis muscle. Use knowledge of anatomy of the musculoskeletal system to answer the question. This will direct you to option 2. Review this anatomic location site for intramuscular injections if you had difficulty with this question.

Level of Cognitive Ability: Application
Client Needs: Safe and Effective Care Environment
Integrated Process: Nursing Process/Implementation
Content Area: Safety and Infection Control

Reference
Harkreader H, Hogan MA: *Fundamentals of nursing: caring and clinical judgment,* ed 2, Philadelphia, 2004, Saunders, p 429.

Multiple Response

14. A nurse manager provides an educational session to nursing staff about client confidentiality. The nurse manager explains that which of the following indicates a breach in client confidentiality? Select all that apply.

   ❏ 1 Leaving a client's medical record in a conference room unattended
   ❏ 2 Providing the client's wife with information about the results of a diagnostic study
   ❏ 3 Placing only a hospital room number on the cover of a hospitalized client's medical record
   ❏ 4 Allowing a student nurse to review diagnostic test results in a client's medical record if the client provides permission to do so
   ❏ 5 Asking the client for written permission for a research team to review his or her medical record
   ❏ 6 Allowing another staff member to use one's computer access code to document vital signs and intake and output amounts

Answer: 1, 2, 6

Rationale: All client information, including medical records, must be kept confidential unless the client has provided written consent to share that information. This includes reading medical records by student nurses or research teams. Medical records cannot be copied or forwarded to anyone, including insurance companies, unless written consent from the client is obtained. Confidentiality even includes preventing family members or friends of the client from acquiring health care information. In the case of computer access, an employee should never provide a computer access code to another person. The nurse needs to protect the client from any breaches in confidentiality; leaving a client's medical record unattended is a breach in confidentiality because it provides an opportunity for others to read client information without the client's consent. Placing only a hospital room number on the cover of a hospitalized client's medical record protects the client because it does not provide public information about the fact that the client is hospitalized. Usually the client is asked to sign written consent or indicate his or her wishes with regard to confidentiality on admission to the hospital or at a physician's office visit.

Test-Taking Strategy: Focus on the subject, situations that indicate a breach in confidentiality. Recalling that a primary nursing responsibility is to protect the client and maintain confidentiality will assist in eliminating options 3, 4, and 5. Review the issues surrounding confidentiality if you had difficulty with this question.

Level of Cognitive Ability: Application
Client Needs: Safe and Effective Care Environment
Integrated Process: Teaching and Learning
Content Area: Management of Care

References
Harkreader H, Hogan MA: *Fundamentals of nursing: caring and clinical judgment,* ed 2, Philadelphia, 2004, Saunders, pp 222-223.
Potter P, Perry A: *Fundamentals of nursing,* ed 6, St Louis, 2005, Mosby, pp 391-392.

Prioritizing (Ordered Response)

15. A nurse manager is planning a teaching session for nursing assistants to reinforce the principles of hand washing. Select in order of priority the steps of the teaching process that the nurse manager should implement. (Number 1 is the first step and number 6 is the last step.)

___ Identify the learning needs of the nursing assistants.

___ Determine achievement of outcomes on the basis of meeting learning objectives.

___ Implement teaching methods involving the nursing assistants in the learning process.

___ Collect and analyze data about the nursing assistants' knowledge of the procedure for hand washing.

___ Prepare a teaching plan identifying learning objectives and the type(s) of teaching methods to be used.

___ Reassess the nursing assistants' ability to perform the skill of hand washing and determine if further teaching is necessary.

Answer: 2, 5, 4, 1, 3, 6

Rationale: The first step of the teaching process includes collecting and analyzing data about the learners' knowledge. The nurse next takes these data and identifies specific learning needs. Once learning needs are determined, the nurse prepares a teaching plan that identifies learning objectives, priorities regarding learning needs, and the teaching methods to be used. The nurse then implements the teaching plan and actively involves the learners. Once teaching is implemented, the nurse evaluates the effectiveness of the plan by determining achievement of outcomes on the basis of meeting learning objectives. Finally, the nurse reassesses knowledge and determines if further teaching in necessary.

Test-Taking Strategy: Focus on the subject, the steps of the teaching process. Use the steps of the nursing process as a guide in determining the correct order of action. Review the steps of the teaching process if you had difficulty with this question.

Level of Cognitive Ability: Application
Client Needs: Safe and Effective Care Environment
Integrated Process: Teaching and Learning
Content Area: Management of Care

References

Harkreader H, Hogan MA: *Fundamentals of nursing: caring and clinical judgment,* ed 2, Philadelphia, 2004, Saunders, p 261.
Potter P, Perry A: *Fundamentals of nursing,* ed 6, St Louis, 2005, Mosby, p 460.

Chart/Exhibit with a Multiple Response

16. A hospitalized client is found lying on the floor next to the bed. Once the client is cared for, the nurse completes an incident (irregular occurrence) report. Select the written statements that identify incorrect documentation on the report.

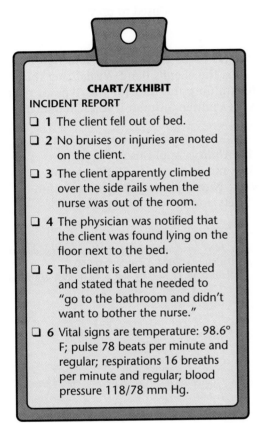

CHART/EXHIBIT
INCIDENT REPORT

❑ **1** The client fell out of bed.

❑ **2** No bruises or injuries are noted on the client.

❑ **3** The client apparently climbed over the side rails when the nurse was out of the room.

❑ **4** The physician was notified that the client was found lying on the floor next to the bed.

❑ **5** The client is alert and oriented and stated that he needed to "go to the bathroom and didn't want to bother the nurse."

❑ **6** Vital signs are temperature: 98.6° F; pulse 78 beats per minute and regular; respirations 16 breaths per minute and regular; blood pressure 118/78 mm Hg.

Answer: 1, 3

Rationale: An incident or irregular occurrence report is a tool used by health care facilities to document situations that have caused harm or have the potential to cause harm to clients, employees, or visitors. The nurse who identifies the situation initiates the report. The report identifies the people involved in the incident, including witnesses; describes the event; and records the date, time, location, factual findings, actions taken, and any other relevant information. The physician is notified of the incident and completes the report after examining the client. Documentation on the report should always be as factual as possible and needs to avoid accusations. Since the client was found lying on the floor, it is unknown whether the client actually fell out of bed. Additionally, the nurse does not know that the client climbed over the side rails when the nurse was out of the room.

Test-Taking Strategy: Focus on the subject, incorrect documentation on the incident report. Recalling that documentation on the report should always be as factual as possible and needs to avoid accusations will assist in answering this question. Review documentation guidelines if you had difficulty with this question.

Level of Cognitive Ability: Analysis
Client Needs: Safe and Effective Care Environment
Integrated Process: Communication and Documentation
Content Area: Safety and Infection Control

Reference
Harkreader H, Hogan MA: *Fundamentals of nursing: caring and clinical judgment,* ed 2, Philadelphia, 2004, Saunders, p 38.

Figure/Illustration with a Multiple Response

17. The nurse would use this type of restraint (refer to figure) in which of the following situations? Select all that apply.

   ❑ 1 To secure the shoulders and the waist
   ❑ 2 To immobilize a client's arm and shoulders
   ❑ 3 To prevent the client from getting out of bed
   ❑ 4 To prevent dislodgement of an intravenous line
   ❑ 5 To prevent the client from turning from side to side
   ❑ 6 To prevent the use of the hands while allowing free arm movement

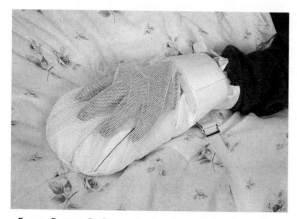

From Potter P, Perry A: *Fundamentals of nursing,* ed 6, St Louis, 2005, Mosby.

Answer: 4, 6

Rationale: A mitten restraint is a thumbless mitten device used to restrain the hands. It prevents the use of the hands while allowing free arm movements. It is useful for a client who needs to be prevented from dislodging an intravenous line, an indwelling urinary catheter, a nasogastric tube or other tubes, or a wound dressing. A jacket restraint or a belt restraint prevents the client from getting out of bed or a chair. A jacket restraint also secures both the shoulders and the waist. A mitten restraint is not used to prevent the client from turning side to side.

Test-Taking Strategy: Focus on the figure and note that it is a device that covers the client's hand. Visualizing this device will assist in determining the uses for this type of restraint. Review the uses for a mitten restraint if you had difficulty with this question.

Level of Cognitive Ability: Application
Client Needs: Safe and Effective Care Environment
Integrated Process: Nursing Process/Implementation
Content Area: Safety and Infection Control

References

Harkreader H, Hogan MA: *Fundamentals of nursing: caring and clinical judgment,* ed 2, Philadelphia, 2004, Saunders, p 510.
Potter P, Perry A: *Fundamentals of nursing,* ed 6, St Louis, 2005, Mosby, p 986.

Multiple Response

18. A home care nurse is visiting an older client who has been recovering from a mild brain attack (stroke) affecting the left side. The client lives alone but receives regular assistance from her daughter and son, who both live within 10 miles. To assess for risk factors related to safety, the nurse should do which of the following? Select all that apply.

❑ **1** Assess the client's visual acuity.

❑ **2** Observe the client's gait and posture.

❑ **3** Evaluate the client's muscle strength.

❑ **4** Look for any hazards in the home care environment.

❑ **5** Ask a family member to move in with the client until recovery is complete.

❑ **6** Request that the client transfer to an assisted living environment for at least 1 month.

Answer: 1, 2, 3, 4

Rationale: To conduct a thorough client assessment, the nurse assesses for possible risk factors related to safety. The assessment should include assessing visual acuity, gait and posture, and muscle strength because alterations in these areas place the client at risk for falls and injury. The nurse should also assess the home environment, looking for any hazards or obstacles that would affect safety. Asking a family member to move in with the client until recovery is complete and requesting that the client transfer to an assisted living environment for at least 1 month are not assessment activities. Additionally, nothing in the question indicates that these actions are necessary; therefore, these options are unrealistic and unreasonable.

Test-Taking Strategy: Focus on the subject, assessing for risk factors related to safety. Note that options 5 and 6 are unrelated to the subject of the question. Review the items that should be included in a safety assessment if you had difficulty with this question.

Level of Cognitive Ability: Application
Client Needs: Safe and Effective Care Environment
Integrated Process: Nursing Process/Assessment
Content Area: Safety and Infection Control

Reference
Potter P, Perry A: *Fundamentals of nursing,* ed 6, St Louis, 2005, Mosby, p 968.

Multiple Response

19. A nurse is reviewing general injury prevention information with the staff of the pediatric department in the hospital. Identify the interventions that the nurse should review to promote safety specifically for infants and toddlers. Select all that apply.

   ❑ 1 Ensure that crib sides are up.
   ❑ 2 Place large, soft pillows in the crib.
   ❑ 3 Use large, soft toys without small parts.
   ❑ 4 Attach a pacifier to a stretchable piece of ribbon and pin to the infant's clothing.
   ❑ 5 Ensure that an infant or toddler is never left unattended while lying on a changing table.
   ❑ 6 Allow a toddler who is toilet training to stay in the bathroom alone to provide privacy.

Answer: 1, 3, 5

Rationale: To promote safety for infants and toddlers, crib sides should never be left down because the child could roll and fall. For this same reason, an infant or toddler is never left unattended while lying on a changing table. Pillows, stuffed toys, comforters, or other objects should not be placed in the crib because the child can become entwined in these items and suffocate. Large, soft toys without small parts should be used because small parts can become dislodged and choking and aspiration may occur. Pacifiers should not be attached to string or ribbon because of the risk associated with choking. The child is never left alone in the bathroom, in the tub, or near any other water source because of the risk of drowning.

Test-Taking Strategy: Focus on the subject, safety measures specific for infants and toddlers. Read each option carefully, thinking about the subject of the question and how the intervention may present a risk to the child. This will assist in answering correctly. Review interventions to ensure safety for infants and toddlers if you had difficulty with this question.

Level of Cognitive Ability: Application
Client Needs: Safe and Effective Care Environment
Integrated Process: Teaching and Learning
Content Area: Safety and Infection Control

Reference
Potter P, Perry A: *Fundamentals of nursing,* ed 6, St Louis, 2005, Mosby, p 977.

Multiple Response

20. Which of the following are accurate principles of sterile technique? Select all that apply.

❏ **1** The edge of a sterile field and 1 to 2 inches inward is unsterile.

❏ **2** If a package is not labeled sterile, it should be considered an unsterile item.

❏ **3** Sterile objects that come in contact with unsterile objects are considered contaminated.

❏ **4** Any part of a sterile field that hangs below the top of the table is sterile as long as it is not touched.

❏ **5** When a sterile field becomes wet, it remains sterile as long as the items on the field are not contaminated.

❏ **6** Items in a sterile package must be used immediately once it has been opened; otherwise it is considered contaminated.

Answer: 1, 2, 3, 6

Rationale: Sterile means the absence of all microorganisms. To maintain sterile technique, the nurse must follow several principles, including the edge of a sterile field and 1 to 2 inches inward is unsterile; sterile packages are labeled as sterile and, if the package is not so labeled, it is considered unsterile; sterile objects that come in contact with unsterile objects are considered contaminated; any part of a sterile field that falls or hangs below the top of the table is unsterile; a sterile field that becomes wet will draw microorganisms from the surface underneath (strike-through) and contaminate the field; and items in a sterile package must be used immediately once it has been opened or it is considered contaminated.

Test-Taking Strategy: Focus on the subject, the accurate principles of sterile technique. Visualize each of the options and think about the principles of sterility to assist in answering the question. Review these principles if you had difficulty with this question.

Level of Cognitive Ability: Comprehension
Client Needs: Safe and Effective Care Environment
Integrated Process: Nursing Process/Implementation
Content Area: Safety and Infection Control

References
Harkreader H, Hogan MA: *Fundamentals of nursing: caring and clinical judgment,* ed 2, Philadelphia, 2004, Saunders, p 476.
Potter P, Perry A: *Fundamentals of nursing,* ed 6, St Louis, 2005, Mosby, p 803.

Multiple Response

21. Which of the following examples relate to medical asepsis to reduce and prevent the spread of microorganisms? Select all that apply.

- ❑ **1** Practicing hand hygiene
- ❑ **2** Reapplying a sterile dressing
- ❑ **3** Sterilizing contaminated items
- ❑ **4** Applying a sterile gown and gloves
- ❑ **5** Routinely cleaning the hospital environment
- ❑ **6** Wearing clean gloves to prevent direct contact with blood or body fluids

Answer: 1, 5, 6

Rationale: Medical asepsis, or clean technique, includes procedures to reduce and prevent the spread of microorganisms. Practicing hand hygiene, wearing clean gloves to prevent direct contact with blood or body fluids, and routinely cleaning the hospital environment are examples of medical asepsis. Surgical asepsis involves the use of sterile technique. Examples of surgical asepsis include reapplying a sterile dressing, sterilization of contaminated items, and applying a sterile gown and gloves.

Test-Taking Strategy: Focus on the subject, medical asepsis. Recalling the definition of medical asepsis and that it involves clean techniques will assist in answering this question. Also note the words *sterile* in options 2 and 4 and the word *sterilizing* in option 3; these words indicate surgical asepsis. Review the difference between medical and surgical asepsis if you had difficulty with this question.

Level of Cognitive Ability: Application
Client Needs: Safe and Effective Care Environment
Integrated Process: Nursing Process/Implementation
Content Area: Safety and Infection Control

Reference

Potter P, Perry A: *Fundamentals of nursing,* ed 6, St Louis, 2005, Mosby, p 788, 802.

Fill-in-the-Blank

22. A physician orders 1000 mL of $^1/_2$% normal saline solution to run over 8 hours. The drop factor is 15 drops/mL. The nurse plans to adjust the flow rate to how many drops per minute to safely administer this intravenous (IV) solution? (Round answer to the nearest whole number.)

Answer: _____ **drops/min**

Answer: 31

Rationale: The prescribed 1000 mL is to be infused over 8 hours. Follow the formula for calculating IV flow rates and multiply 1000 mL by 15 (drop factor). Then divide the result by 480 minutes (8 hours × 60 minutes). The infusion is to run at 31.2 or 31 drops/min.

Formula

$$\frac{\text{Total volume in mL} \times \text{Drop factor}}{\text{Time in minutes}} = \text{Flow rate in drops/min}$$

$$\frac{1000 \text{ mL} \times 15 \text{ drops/mL}}{480 \text{ min}} = \frac{15,000}{480} = 31.2 \text{ or } 31 \text{ drops/min}$$

Test-Taking Strategy: Follow the formula for calculating the infusion rate for an IV and be certain to change 8 hours to 480 minutes. After you have performed the calculation, verify your answer using a calculator. Review the formula for safely calculating infusion rates if you had difficulty with this question.

Level of Cognitive Ability: Application
Client Needs: Safe and Effective Care Environment
Integrated Process: Nursing Process/Implementation
Content Area: Safety and Infection Control

Reference

Kee J, Marshall S: *Clinical calculations: with applications to general and specialty areas*, ed 5, Philadelphia, 2004, Saunders, p 202.

Chart/Exhibit with a Multiple Response

23. At the scene of a train crash, the nurse triages the victims. Which clients would be coded for triage as most urgent or the first priority? Select all that apply.

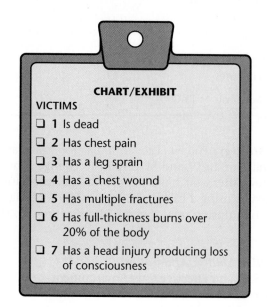

CHART/EXHIBIT

VICTIMS

❏ **1** Is dead

❏ **2** Has chest pain

❏ **3** Has a leg sprain

❏ **4** Has a chest wound

❏ **5** Has multiple fractures

❏ **6** Has full-thickness burns over 20% of the body

❏ **7** Has a head injury producing loss of consciousness

Answer: 2, 4, 6, 7

Rationale: In a disaster situation, saving the greatest number of lives is the most important goal. During a disaster the nurse would triage the victims to maximize the number of survivors and sort the treatable from the untreatable victims. Prioritizing victims can be done in many ways, and many communities use a color coding system. First priority victims (most urgent and coded red) have life-threatening injuries and are experiencing hypoxia or near hypoxia. Examples of injuries in this category are shock, chest wounds, internal hemorrhage, head injuries producing loss of consciousness, partial- or full-thickness burns over 20% to 60% of the body surface, and chest pain. Second priority victims (urgent and coded yellow) have injuries with systemic effects but are not yet hypoxic or in shock and can withstand a 2-hour wait without immediate risk (e.g., a victim with multiple fractures). Third priority victims (coded green) have minimal injuries unaccompanied by systemic complications and can wait for more than 2 hours for treatment without risk (leg sprain). Dying or dead victims have catastrophic injuries, and the dying victims would not survive under the best of circumstances (coded black).

Test-Taking Strategy: Focus on the subject, the victims of a disaster that are most urgent or the first priority. Read each option carefully and recall that in a disaster situation, saving the greatest number of lives is the most important goal and that the nurse would triage the victims to maximize the number of survivors. Also, use of the ABCs (airway, breathing, and circulation) will direct you to the correct options. Review triage systems for disasters if you had difficulty with this question.

Level of Cognitive Ability: Analysis
Client Needs: Safe and Effective Care Environment
Integrated Process: Nursing Process/Assessment
Content Area: Management of Care

Reference
Maurer F, Smith C: *Community public health nursing practice: health for families and populations,* ed 3, Philadelphia, 2005, Saunders, pp 505-506.

Chart/Exhibit with a Multiple Response

24. The physician writes medication orders at 9 AM on February 9, 2008, for an adult client and signs the orders. Which order(s) should the nurse question? Select all that apply.

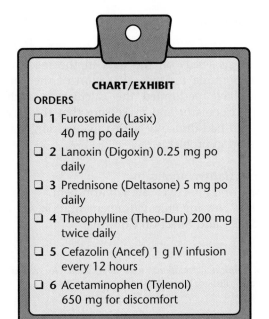

CHART/EXHIBIT

ORDERS

❑ **1** Furosemide (Lasix)
    40 mg po daily

❑ **2** Lanoxin (Digoxin) 0.25 mg po
    daily

❑ **3** Prednisone (Deltasone) 5 mg po
    daily

❑ **4** Theophylline (Theo-Dur) 200 mg
    twice daily

❑ **5** Cefazolin (Ancef) 1 g IV infusion
    every 12 hours

❑ **6** Acetaminophen (Tylenol)
    650 mg for discomfort

Answer: 4, 6

Rationale: The basic components of a medication order are the date and time that the order was written, medication name, medication dosage, route of administration, frequency of administration, and the physician's signature. If any of these components is missing, the nurse contacts the physician to question the order. Order 4, theophylline, is incomplete because it is missing the route. Order 6, acetaminophen, is incomplete because it is missing the route and frequency.

Test-Taking Strategy: Focus on the subject, the medication orders that the nurse should question. This indicates that you are identifying the orders that are inaccurate or incomplete. Recalling that medication orders need to contain the medication dosage, route of administration, and frequency of administration will assist in answering this question. Review the basic components of a medication order if you had difficulty with this question.

Level of Cognitive Ability: Application
Client Needs: Safe and Effective Care Environment
Integrated Process: Nursing Process/Implementation
Content Area: Safety and Infection Control

Reference
Kee J, Marshall S: *Clinical calculations: with applications to general and specialty areas,* ed 5, Philadelphia, 2004, Saunders, p 52.

Figure/Illustration with a Fill-in-the-Blank

25. The physician prescribes amoxicillin (Amoxil) 500 mg liquid orally every 8 hours. The nurse prepares how many milliliters to safely administer one dose? (Refer to figure.)

Answer: _____ mL

Answer: 20

Rationale: Use the medication calculation formula.

Formula

$$\frac{\text{Desired} \times \text{mL}}{\text{Available}} = \text{mL/dose}$$

$$\frac{500 \text{ mg} \times 5 \text{ mL}}{125 \text{ mg}} = 20 \text{ mL/dose}$$

Test-Taking Strategy: Focus on the data in the medication label. Follow the formula for the calculation of the correct dose. Once you have performed the calculation, recheck your work with a calculator and make sure that the answer makes sense. If you had difficulty with this question, review medication calculation problems.

Level of Cognitive Ability: Application
Client Needs: Safe and Effective Care Environment
Integrated Process: Nursing Process/Implementation
Content Area: Safety and Infection Control

Reference
Kee J, Marshall S: *Clinical calculations: with applications to general and specialty areas,* ed 5, Philadelphia, 2004, Saunders, p 80.

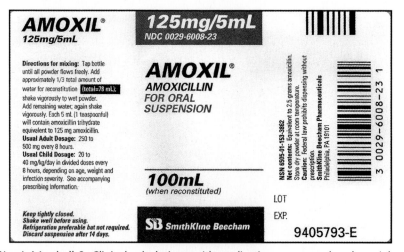

From Kee J, Marshall S: *Clinical calculations: with applications to general and specialty areas,* ed 5, Philadelphia, 2004, Saunders.

Prioritizing (Ordered Response)

26. List in order of priority how the nurse should best schedule morning activities for assigned clients. (Number 1 is the first activity and number 6 is the last activity.)

_____ Make rounds and assess assigned clients.

_____ Receive report from the previous nursing shift.

_____ Administer medications scheduled before breakfast.

_____ Perform daily dressing changes and other treatments.

_____ Document nursing care and other pertinent information in the client's record.

_____ Ensure that clients receive breakfast and receive hygiene care by the nursing assistant.

Answer: 2, 1, 3, 5, 6, 4

Rationale: Time management and organization require the nurse to identify tasks, obligations, and activities that must be accomplished in a given period. Based on the activities listed, the nurse first receives report from the previous shift to identify client needs. The nurse next makes rounds and assesses assigned clients. This is an important activity that needs to be performed early in the shift to obtain a baseline measure of the client's condition that can be reassessed throughout the shift. Additionally, if the client's condition changes during the shift, the nurse has a baseline assessment for comparison. The nurse next administers medications scheduled before meals and then ensures that clients receive breakfast and receive hygiene care by the nursing assistant. The nurse performs treatments prescribed in addition to administering any other scheduled midmorning medications. Finally, the nurse documents nursing care and other pertinent information.

Test-Taking Strategy: Focus on the subject, how the nurse should best schedule morning activities for assigned clients. Read each of the activities listed and think about your clinical experiences and how activities were planned. Remember that it is necessary to receive report from the previous shift and assess assigned clients. Also remember that, although the nurse should be documenting on his or her worksheet throughout the shift, documenting of care and any other pertinent information is usually the last activity and is done once client care is complete and client needs are met. Review time management skills if you had difficulty with this question.

Level of Cognitive Ability: Application
Client Needs: Safe and Effective Care Environment
Integrated Process: Nursing Process/Planning
Content Area: Management of Care

Reference
Harkreader H, Hogan MA: *Fundamentals of nursing: caring and clinical judgment,* ed 2, Philadelphia, 2004, Saunders, p 281.

Multiple Response

27. A nurse manager is reviewing infection control interventions with the nursing staff and tells the staff that which of these interventions will reduce reservoirs of infection? Select all that apply.

   ❏ 1 Keeping bedside table surfaces clean and dry
   ❏ 2 Placing tissues and soiled dressings in paper bags
   ❏ 3 Changing dressings that become wet or soiled
   ❏ 4 Placing capped needles and syringes in puncture-resistant containers
   ❏ 5 Using soap and water to remove drainage, dried secretions, or excess perspiration from the client's skin
   ❏ 6 Emptying urinary drainage systems (Foley catheter drainage) on each shift unless otherwise ordered by a physician

Answer: 1, 3, 5, 6

Rationale: Infection control measures to reduce reservoirs of infection include keeping bedside table surfaces clean and dry; placing tissues, soiled dressings, or soiled linens in moisture-resistant bags (not paper bags); changing dressings that become wet or soiled; placing syringes and uncapped needles in puncture-resistant containers; using soap and water to remove drainage, dried secretions, or excess perspiration from the client's skin; and emptying all drainage systems on each shift unless otherwise ordered by a physician.

Test-Taking Strategy: Focus on the subject, interventions that will reduce reservoirs of infection. Read each option carefully and eliminate option 2 because of the word *paper* and option 4 because of the word *capped*. Review interventions that will reduce reservoirs of infection if you had difficulty with this question.

Level of Cognitive Ability: Application
Client Needs: Safe and Effective Care Environment
Integrated Process: Teaching and Learning
Content Area: Safety and Infection Control

Reference
Potter P, Perry A: *Fundamentals of nursing*, ed 6, St Louis, 2005, Mosby, p 789.

Multiple Response

28. The nurse is preparing the client assignment for the day and needs to assign clients to a licensed practical nurse (LPN) and a nursing assistant. Which clients should the nurse assign to the LPN because of client needs that cannot be met by the nursing assistant? Select all that apply.

   ❏ 1 A client requiring frequent suctioning
   ❏ 2 A client requiring a dressing change to the foot
   ❏ 3 A client requiring range-of-motion exercises twice daily
   ❏ 4 A client requiring reinforcement of teaching about a diabetic diet
   ❏ 5 A client on bed rest requiring vital sign measurement every 4 hours
   ❏ 6 A client requiring collection of a urine specimen for urinalysis testing

Answer: 1, 2, 4

Rationale: Delegation is the transferring to a competent individual the authority to perform a nursing task. When the nurse plans client assignments, he or she needs to consider the educational level of the individual and the needs of the client. The LPN is trained to perform all the tasks indicated in the options; the clients who have needs that cannot be met by the nursing assistant are those requiring suctioning, a dressing change, and reinforcement of teaching about a diabetic diet. A nursing assistant is trained to perform range-of-motion exercises, measure vital signs, and collect a urine specimen.

Test-Taking Strategy: Focus on the subject, client needs that cannot be met by the nursing assistant. Read each option carefully and consider the needs of the client. Recalling that the nursing assistant can be assigned activities that are non-invasive will assist in answering the question. Review the principles related to delegation if you had difficulty with this question.

Level of Cognitive Ability: Application
Client Needs: Safe and Effective Care Environment
Integrated Process: Nursing Process/Planning
Content Area: Management of Care

References
Harkreader H, Hogan MA: *Fundamentals of nursing: caring and clinical judgment,* ed 2, Philadelphia, 2004, Saunders, p 282.
Huber D: *Leadership and nursing care management,* ed 3, Philadelphia, 2006, Saunders, p 544.

Multiple Response

29. A nurse manager is providing an educational session to the nursing staff in a skilled nursing facility on the guidelines for the safe use of physical restraints. Which of the following are safe guidelines? Select all that apply.

❏ **1** A physician's order is required.
❏ **2** Restraints should be secured with a quick-release tie.
❏ **3** Restraints are secured to side rails so that they can be easily removed as necessary.
❏ **4** Restraints are used only when other measures have failed to prevent self-injury or injury to others.
❏ **5** Restraints can be used as a usual part of treatment plans, as indicated by the client's condition or symptoms.
❏ **6** The use of restraints can be ordered prn (as needed) as long as the nurse performs a thorough assessment before applying them.

Answer: 1, 2, 4

Rationale: A physical restraint is a mechanical or physical device that is used to immobilize a client or extremity. They restrict the freedom of movement or normal access to a client's body. A physician's order is required for the use of restraints. Restraints are not a usual part of treatment plans, indicated by the person's condition or symptoms, and are not prescribed on a prn basis. Restraints are considered for use only when other measures have failed to prevent self-injury or injury to others. Restraints should be secured with a quick-release tie so that they can be easily removed in an emergency. Restraints are secured to the bed frame, not the side rails, because the client may be injured if the side rail is lowered.

Test-Taking Strategy: Focus on the subject, guidelines for the safe use of physical restraints. Read each option and carefully think about two issues: client safety and the legalities related to the use of restraints. This will assist in answering the question. Review these guidelines if you had difficulty with this question.

Level of Cognitive Ability: Application
Client Needs: Safe and Effective Care Environment
Integrated Process: Teaching and Learning
Content Area: Safety and Infection Control

Reference
Potter P, Perry A: *Fundamentals of nursing*, ed 6, St Louis, 2005, Mosby, pp 411, 980-981.

Multiple Response

30. An emergency department nurse is a member of an All-Hazards Disaster Preparedness planning group. The group is developing a specific emergency response plan in the event that a client with smallpox arrives in the emergency department. Select all interventions that should be included in the plan.

❑ **1** Isolate the client.
❑ **2** Don protective equipment immediately.
❑ **3** Lock down the emergency department and the entire hospital immediately.
❑ **4** Notify infectious disease specialists, public health officials, and the police.
❑ **5** Identify all client contacts, including transport services to the emergency department and clients in the waiting room.
❑ **6** Administer smallpox vaccines to all hospital staff, client contacts, and clients sitting in the emergency department waiting room immediately.

Answer: 1, 2, 4, 5

Rationale: An All-Hazards Disaster Preparedness group is a multifaceted internal and external disaster preparedness group that establishes action plans for every type of disaster or combination of disaster events. In the event of emergency department exposure to a communicable disease such as smallpox, the client would be isolated immediately and the staff would immediately don protective equipment. The emergency department would be locked down immediately. Infectious disease specialists and public health officials will determine whether it is necessary to lock down the entire hospital. Infectious disease specialists, public health officials, and the police are notified. All client contacts (name, addresses, telephone numbers), including transport services to the emergency department and clients in the waiting room, would be identified so that the public health department can follow through on notifying and treating these individuals appropriately. Although getting the vaccine within 3 days after exposure will help prevent the disease or make it less severe, it is unreasonable and unnecessary to administer smallpox vaccines to all hospital staff, client contacts, and clients sitting in the emergency department waiting room.

Test-Taking Strategy: Focus on the subject, a client with smallpox in the emergency department. Next read each option carefully, noting that the client is in the emergency department. Eliminate option 3 because of the words *entire hospital* and option 6 because of the words *all hospital staff*. Review disaster preparedness if you had difficulty with this question.

Level of Cognitive Ability: Application
Client Needs: Safe and Effective Care Environment
Integrated Process: Nursing Process/Planning
Content Area: Safety and Infection Control

Reference
Huber D: *Leadership and nursing care management,* ed 3, Philadelphia, 2006, Saunders, p 451.

Multiple Response

31. A deceased client with multiple gunshot wounds arrives by ambulance to the emergency department. The nurse is caring for the client's personal belongings, which may be needed as legal evidence. Which actions should the nurse take to properly secure and handle legal evidence? Select all that apply.

   ❑ 1 Place paper bags on the hands and feet.
   ❑ 2 Give the clothing and wallet to the family.
   ❑ 3 Cut clothing along the seams, avoiding bullet holes.
   ❑ 4 Collect all personal items, including items from clothing pockets.
   ❑ 5 Place wet clothing and personal belongings in a labeled, sealed plastic bag.
   ❑ 6 Do not allow family members, significant others, or friends to be alone with the client.

Answer: 1, 3, 4, 6

Rationale: Basic rules for securing and handling evidence include minimally handling the body of a deceased person; placing paper bags on the hands and feet and possibly over the head of a deceased person (protects trace evidence and residue); placing clothing and personal items in paper bags (plastic bags can destroy items because items can sweat in plastic); cutting clothes along seams, avoiding areas where there are obvious holes or tears; and collecting all personal items, including items from clothing pockets. Evidence is never released to the family to take home, and family members, significant others, or friends are not allowed to be alone with the client because of the possibility of jeopardizing any existing legal evidence.

Test-Taking Strategy: Focus on the subject, proper securing and handling of legal evidence. Read each option carefully and visualize and think about how the action may or may not preserve evidence. This strategy will direct you to the correct actions. If this question was difficult, review the basic rules for securing and handling evidence.

Level of Cognitive Ability: Application
Client Needs: Safe and Effective Care Environment
Integrated Process: Nursing Process/Implementation
Content Area: Fundamental Skills

Reference
Black J, Hawks J: *Medical-surgical nursing: clinical management for positive outcomes,* ed 7, Philadelphia, 2005, Saunders, p 2483.

Prioritizing (Ordered Response)

32. Select the order of action that the nurse takes to perform hand-washing procedure. (Number 1 is the first action and number 6 is the last action.)

_____ Dry the hands.

_____ Turn off the water faucet.

_____ Rinse the hands and wrists.

_____ Wash all surfaces for 15 to 30 seconds.

_____ Obtain 3 to 5 mL of soap from the dispenser.

_____ Wet the hands and wrists, keeping the hands lower than the elbows.

Answer: 5, 6, 4, 3, 2, 1

Rationale: Proper hand-washing procedure involves wetting the hands and wrists and keeping the hands lower than the forearms so water flows toward the fingertips. The nurse uses 3 to 5 mL of soap and washes all surfaces for 15 to 30 seconds using a rubbing and circular motion. The hands are rinsed and then dried, moving from the fingers to the forearms. The paper towel is then discarded, and a second one is used to turn off the faucet to avoid hand contamination.

Test-Taking Strategy: Focus on the subject, the order of action that the nurse takes to perform hand-washing procedure. Visualizing this procedure will assist in determining the correct order of action. Review this fundamental nursing procedure if you had difficulty with this question.

Level of Cognitive Ability: Application
Client Needs: Safe and Effective Care Environment
Integrated Process: Nursing Process/Implementation
Content Area: Safety and Infection Control

Reference
Harkreader H, Hogan MA: *Fundamentals of nursing: caring and clinical judgment,* ed 2, Philadelphia, 2004, Saunders, pp 465-466.

Multiple Response

33. A client who is immunosuppressed is being admitted to the hospital on neutropenic precautions. Nursing interventions to protect the client from infection include which measures? Select all that apply.

- ❏ **1** Restrict all visitors.
- ❏ **2** Admit the client to a semiprivate room.
- ❏ **3** Place a mask on the client if the client leaves the room.
- ❏ **4** Use strict aseptic technique for all invasive procedures.
- ❏ **5** Place a "See the Nurse before Entering" sign on the door to the room.
- ❏ **6** Remove a vase with fresh flowers in the room that was left by a previous client.

Answer: 3, 4, 5, 6

Rationale: The client who is on neutropenic precautions is immunosuppressed and therefore is admitted to a single room on the nursing unit. A sign indicating "See the Nurse before Entering" should be placed on the door to the client's room so the nurse can ensure that neutropenic precautions are implemented by anyone entering the room. Sources of standing water and fresh flowers should be removed to decrease the microorganism count. The client should wear a mask for protection from exposure to microorganisms whenever he or she leaves the room. Not all visitors need to be restricted; however, visitors need to be restricted to healthy adults and need to perform strict hand-washing procedures and don a mask before entering the client's room. The use of strict aseptic technique is necessary with all invasive procedures to prevent infection.

Test-Taking Strategy: Focus on the subject, an immunosuppressed client and neutropenic precautions. Read each option carefully and recall that the client is at risk for contracting infection. Select the options that protect the client from infection. Review this type of infection control precaution if you had difficulty with this question.

Level of Cognitive Ability: Application
Client Needs: Safe and Effective Care Environment
Integrated Process: Nursing Process/Implementation
Content Area: Safety and Infection Control

References
Black J, Hawks J: *Medical-surgical nursing: clinical management for positive outcomes,* ed 7, Philadelphia, 2005, Saunders, p 382.
Ignatavicius D, Workman M: *Medical surgical nursing: critical thinking for collaborative care,* ed 5, Philadelphia, 2006, Saunders, p 497.

Multiple Response

34. A client receiving chemotherapy has an extremely low white blood cell count and is immediately placed on neutropenic precautions that includes a low-bacteria diet. Which food items is the client allowed to consume? Select all that apply.

- ❑ **1** Fresh apple
- ❑ **2** Raw celery
- ❑ **3** Italian bread
- ❑ **4** Tossed salad
- ❑ **5** Baked chicken
- ❑ **6** Well-done (well-cooked) cheeseburger

Answer: 3, 5, 6

Rationale: An extremely low white blood cell count places the client at risk for infection. In the immunocompromised client, a low-bacteria diet is implemented. This diet includes avoiding fresh fruits and vegetables and ensuring that meat is thoroughly cooked. Fresh fruits and vegetables harbor organisms and place the client at risk for infection. Italian bread, baked chicken, and a well-done cheeseburger are acceptable to consume.

Test-Taking Strategy: Focus on the subject, a low-bacteria diet. Read each option carefully and think about the food items that harbor bacteria. Recalling that fresh fruits and vegetables are restricted from a low-bacteria diet will assist in selecting the correct items. Review interventions for the client on a low-bacteria diet if you had difficulty with this question.

Level of Cognitive Ability: Application
Client Needs: Safe and Effective Care Environment
Integrated Process: Nursing Process/Implementation
Content Area: Safety and Infection Control

References

Black J, Hawks J: *Medical-surgical nursing: clinical management for positive outcomes,* ed 7, Philadelphia, 2005, Saunders, p 2302.
Ignatavicius D, Workman M: *Medical surgical nursing: critical thinking for collaborative care,* ed 5, Philadelphia, 2006, p 497.

Prioritizing (Ordered Response)

35. A nurse has cared for a client on isolation that required the use of gloves, a mask, goggles, and a gown. Select in order of priority how the nurse removes the protective items on leaving the client's room. (Number 1 is the first action and number 6 is the last action.)

    ___ Removes goggles
    ___ Removes the mask
    ___ Removes the gloves
    ___ Allows the gown to fall from the shoulders
    ___ Unties the neck strings and the back strings of the gown
    ___ Holds the gown inside at the shoulder seams, folds it inside out, and discards it in the appropriate trash receptacle or laundry bag

Answer: 6, 2, 1, 4, 3, 5

Rationale: The nurse should remove gloves first because these are the items that are most contaminated. The nurse then carefully removes the mask by touching only the elastic or mask strings. Ungloved hands will not become contaminated by touching only the elastic or mask strings. Then the nurse unties the neck strings and the back strings of the gown and allows the gown to fall from the shoulders. The nurse removes the hands from the sleeves, without touching the outside of the gown, holds the gown inside at the shoulder seams, folds it inside out, and discards it in the appropriate trash receptacle or laundry bag. The nurse removes the goggles and then washes the hands.

Test-Taking Strategy: Use knowledge of Standard Precautions and the methods to prevent contamination and visualize the procedure for removing contaminated clothing and items after caring for a client to assist in determining the correct order of action. Remember that the gloves are the items that are most contaminated and are removed first. Review this procedure if you had difficulty with this question.

Level of Cognitive Ability: Application
Client Needs: Safe and Effective Care Environment
Integrated Process: Nursing Process/Implementation
Content Area: Safety and Infection Control

Reference
Perry A, Potter P: *Clinical nursing skills and techniques,* ed 6, St Louis, 2006, Mosby, p 203.

Prioritizing (Ordered Response)

36. Place in order of priority the steps that the nurse should take in a fire emergency. (Number 1 is the first step and number 6 is the last step.)

___ Contain the fire.
___ Activate the alarm.
___ Pull the pin on the fire extinguisher.
___ Aim the extinguisher at the base of the fire.
___ Remove any victims from the vicinity of the fire.
___ Squeeze the handle and sweep the extinguisher from side to side to coat the area evenly.

Answer: 3, 2, 4, 5, 1, 6

Rationale: In a fire emergency the steps to follow use the acronym RACE: first, *R*emove (or *R*escue) the victim, then *A*ctivate the alarm, *C*ontain the fire, and *E*xtinguish as needed. This is a universal standard that may be applied to any type of fire emergency. The steps to follow to use a fire extinguisher use the acronym PASS: first, pull the *P*in; then *A*im the extinguisher at the base of the fire; and finally *S*queeze the handle of the extinguisher and extinguish the fire by *S*weeping the extinguisher from side to side to coat the area evenly.

Test-Taking Strategy: Focus on the subject of the question, a fire emergency. Sequencing the activities using the RACE and the PASS acronym will determine the correct order of action. Review fire safety if you had difficulty with this question.

Level of Cognitive Ability: Application
Client Needs: Safe and Effective Care Environment
Integrated Process: Nursing Process/Implementation
Content Area: Safety and Infection Control

References

Harkreader H, Hogan MA: *Fundamentals of nursing: caring and clinical judgment*, ed 2, Philadelphia, 2004, Saunders, p 505.
Potter P, Perry A: *Fundamentals of nursing*, ed 6, St Louis, 2005, Mosby, p 992.

Figure/Illustration with a Fill-in-the-Blank

37. The nurse needs to withdraw 7000 units from the medication vial for administration. The nurse withdraws how many milliliters for a safe dose of medication? (Refer to figure.)

Answer: _____ mL

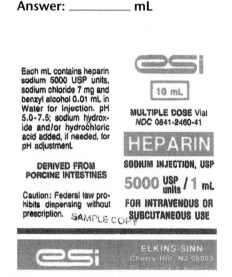

Each mL contains heparin sodium 5000 USP units, sodium chloride 7 mg and benzyl alcohol 0.01 mL in Water for Injection. pH 5.0-7.5; sodium hydroxide and/or hydrochloric acid added, if needed, for pH adjustment.

DERIVED FROM PORCINE INTESTINES

Caution: Federal law prohibits dispensing without prescription. SAMPLE COPY

esi

10 mL

MULTIPLE DOSE Vial
NDC 0641-2460-41

HEPARIN

SODIUM INJECTION, USP

5000 USP units / 1 mL

FOR INTRAVENOUS OR SUBCUTANEOUS USE

esi   ELKINS-SINN
Cherry Hill NJ 08003

From Kee J, Marshall S: *Clinical calculations: with applications to general and specialty areas,* ed 5, Philadelphia, 2004, Saunders.

Answer: 1.4

Rationale: Use the medication calculation formula.

Formula

$$\frac{\text{Desired} \times \text{mL}}{\text{Available}} = \text{mL/dose}$$

$$\frac{7000 \text{ units} \times 1 \text{ mL}}{5000 \text{ units}} = 1.4 \text{ mL/dose}$$

Test-Taking Strategy: Focus on the data in the medication label. Follow the formula for calculating the correct dose. Once you have performed the calculation, recheck your work with a calculator and make certain that the answer makes sense. If you had difficulty with this question, review medication calculation problems.

Level of Cognitive Ability: Application
Client Needs: Safe and Effective Care Environment
Integrated Process: Nursing Process/Implementation
Content Area: Safety and Infection Control

Reference
Kee J, Marshall S: *Clinical calculations: with applications to general and specialty areas,* ed 5, Philadelphia, 2004, Saunders, p 80.

Multiple Response

38. The nurse implements which measures to prevent an electrical shock when using electrical equipment? Select all that apply.

❑ **1** Use a two-prong outlet.
❑ **2** Check the electrical cord for fraying.
❑ **3** Keep the electrical cord away from the sink.
❑ **4** Place the excess electrical cord under a small carpet.
❑ **5** Grasp the electrical cord when unplugging the equipment.
❑ **6** Disconnect the electrical cord from the wall socket when cleaning the equipment.

Answer: 2, 3, 6

Rationale: The nurse needs to implement measures to prevent an electrical shock when using electrical equipment. These measures include using a three-prong plug that is grounded, checking the electrical cord for fraying or other damage, keeping the electrical cord away from the sink or other sources of water, using electrical tape to secure the excess electrical cord to the floor where it will not be stepped on (the cord should not be placed under carpet), grasping the plug (not the electrical cord) when unplugging the equipment, and disconnecting the electrical cord from the wall socket when cleaning the equipment.

Test-Taking Strategy: Focus on the subject, electrical safety. Read each option carefully and visualize how the measure may or may not prevent an electrical shock. If you had difficulty with this question, review the measures that will prevent an electrical shock when using electrical equipment.

Level of Cognitive Ability: Application
Client Needs: Safe and Effective Care Environment
Integrated Process: Nursing Process/Implementation
Content Area: Safety and Infection Control

Reference
Potter P, Perry A: *Fundamentals of nursing,* ed 6, St Louis, 2005, Mosby, p 993.

Multiple Response

39. Which actions will the nurse take in the event of an accidental poisoning? Select all that apply.

❑ **1** Save vomitus for laboratory analysis.

❑ **2** Place the client in a flat supine position.

❑ **3** Induce vomiting if a household cleaner was ingested.

❑ **4** Assess for airway patency, breathing, and circulation.

❑ **5** Determine the type and amount of substance ingested.

❑ **6** Remove any visible materials from the nose and mouth.

Answer: 1, 4, 5, 6

Rationale: In the event of accidental poisoning, the poison control center is called before attempting any interventions. Additional interventions in an accidental poisoning include assess for airway patency, breathing, and circulation; remove any visible materials from the nose and mouth to terminate exposure; determine the type and amount of substance ingested if possible to identify an antidote; save vomitus for laboratory analysis, which may assist with further treatment; and position the victim with the head to the side to prevent aspiration of vomitus and assist in keeping the airway open. Vomiting is never induced in an unconscious client or in a client who is experiencing seizures because of the risk of aspiration. Additionally, vomiting is not induced if lye, household cleaners, hair care products, grease or petroleum products, or furniture polish was ingested because of the risk of internal burns.

Test-Taking Strategy: Focus on the subject, interventions in the event of accidental poisoning. Visualize each of the interventions and how they may be helpful in treating the poisoning. Use of the ABCs (airway, breathing, and circulation) will assist in determining the correct interventions. Also remember that any substances that are caustic can result in further injury to the client. If you had difficulty with this question, review the interventions for treating a victim of accidental poisoning.

Level of Cognitive Ability: Application
Client Needs: Safe and Effective Care Environment
Integrated Process: Nursing Process/Implementation
Content Area: Safety and Infection Control

Reference
Potter P, Perry A: *Fundamentals of nursing*, ed 6, St Louis, 2005, Mosby, p 993.

Multiple Response

40. Which interventions should the emergency department nurse take during the management of a client suspected of exposure to anthrax? Select all that apply.

❑ **1** Handle clothing minimally.
❑ **2** Instruct the client to remove contaminated clothing.
❑ **3** Store contaminated clothing in a labeled paper bag.
❑ **4** Wear sterile gloves when handling contaminated items.
❑ **5** Instruct the client to shower thoroughly using soap and water.
❑ **6** Consult with the physician regarding postexposure prophylaxis with oral fluoroquinolones for the client.

Answer: 1, 2, 5, 6

Rationale: An important aspect of care for a client who has a bioterrorism-related illness is postexposure management. Decontamination and exposure management of the client suspected of anthrax exposure include instructing the client to remove contaminated clothing and store contaminated clothing in a labeled plastic (not paper) bag; handling clothing minimally to avoid agitation; instructing the client to shower thoroughly using soap and water; and using Standard Precautions and wearing appropriate protective barriers when handling contaminated clothing or other items. The use of sterile gloves is unnecessary. Postexposure prophylaxis with oral fluoroquinolones for the client is also recommended.

Test-Taking Strategy: Focus on the subject, a client suspected of exposure to anthrax. Read each option carefully. Recalling that postexposure management involves decontamination will assist in selecting the correct interventions. Remember, preventing exposure is a critical intervention. If you had difficulty with this question, review the interventions for postexposure management of bioterrorist-related illnesses.

Level of Cognitive Ability: Application
Client Needs: Safe and Effective Care Environment
Integrated Process: Nursing Process/Implementation
Content Area: Safety and Infection Control

Reference
Potter P, Perry A: *Fundamentals of nursing,* ed 6, St Louis, 2005, Mosby, p 996.

Chart/Exhibit with a Multiple Response

41. Which clients require contact precautions? Refer to chart/exhibit. Select all that apply.

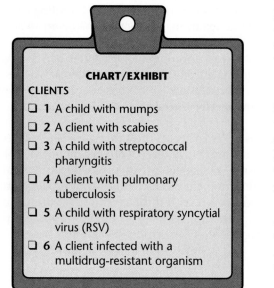

CHART/EXHIBIT

CLIENTS

❑ **1** A child with mumps

❑ **2** A client with scabies

❑ **3** A child with streptococcal pharyngitis

❑ **4** A client with pulmonary tuberculosis

❑ **5** A child with respiratory syncytial virus (RSV)

❑ **6** A client infected with a multidrug-resistant organism

Answer: 2, 5, 6

Rationale: Contact precautions are initiated when disease transmission occurs from direct contact with the client or the client's environment. Diseases that require the use of contact precautions include colonization or infection with multidrug-resistant organisms; RSV; shigella and other enteric pathogens; major wound infections; herpes simplex; scabies; and disseminated varicella zoster. Clients with mumps or streptococcal pharyngitis require droplet precautions. A client with pulmonary tuberculosis requires airborne precautions.

Test-Taking Strategy: Focus on the subject, clients who require contact precautions. Read each client description in the chart/exhibit. Determining the mode of transmission for each illness will assist in answering this question correctly. If you had difficulty with this question, review the modes of transmission for each illness identified and the diseases that require contact precautions.

Level of Cognitive Ability: Application
Client Needs: Safe and Effective Care Environment
Integrated Process: Nursing Process/Implementation
Content Area: Safety and Infection Control

Reference
Potter P, Perry A: *Fundamentals of nursing,* ed 6, St Louis, 2005, Mosby, p 797.

Multiple Response

42. Which of the following are characteristics of team nursing? Select all that apply.

- ❏ **1** Nursing assistants are given a client assignment.
- ❏ **2** A registered nurse leads a team of staff members.
- ❏ **3** Each nurse assumes responsibility for a specific task.
- ❏ **4** Team members provide direct care to groups of clients.
- ❏ **5** The registered nurse assumes responsibility for a caseload of clients over time.
- ❏ **6** Team nursing maintains continuity of care across nursing shifts, days, and home care visits.

Answer: 1, 2, 4

Rationale: In team nursing a registered nurse (RN) leads a team that is composed of other RNs, licensed practical or licensed vocational nurses, and nursing assistants and technicians. The team members provide direct client care to groups of clients under the direct supervision of the RN team leader. In this model, nursing assistants are given client assignments rather than being assigned particular nursing tasks. In functional nursing, tasks are divided, with one nurse assuming responsibility for specific tasks. Primary nursing is a model in which the RN assumes responsibility for a caseload of clients over time. In primary nursing, continuity of care across nursing shifts, days, and home care visits is maintained.

Test-Taking Strategy: Focus on the subject, the characteristics of team nursing. Thinking about the definition of and the concepts related to the word *team* will assist in answering the question. Review the characteristics of team nursing if you had difficulty with this question.

Level of Cognitive Ability: Comprehension
Client Needs: Safe and Effective Care Environment
Integrated Process: Nursing Process/Implementation
Content Area: Management of Care

Reference

Potter P, Perry A: *Fundamentals of nursing*, ed 6, St Louis, 2005, Mosby, p 797.

Multiple Response

43. Which of the following are responsibilities of a nurse manager? Select all that apply.

❑ **1** Recruit new employees.
❑ **2** Conduct regular staff meetings.
❑ **3** Assist staff in meeting annual goals.
❑ **4** Monitor professional standards of practice on the nursing unit.
❑ **5** Expect nursing staff to problem solve all client or family complaints.
❑ **6** Write orders for physicians when conducting rounds with the physicians.

Answer: 1, 2, 3, 4

Rationale: Responsibilities of a nurse manager include recruiting new employees (interviewing and hiring), conducting regular staff meetings, assisting staff in meeting annual goals for the unit and systems needed to accomplish goals, monitoring professional standards of practice on the nursing unit, developing an ongoing staff development plan, conducting routine staff evaluations, acting as a role model, submitting staff schedules for the unit, conducting regular client rounds and problem solving client and family complaints, establishing and implementing a unit quality improvement plan, and conducting rounds with physicians. The nurse is not responsible for writing orders for physicians when conducting rounds; the physician is responsible for writing orders.

Test-Taking Strategy: Focus on the subject, the responsibilities of a nurse manager. Recalling that a nurse manager functions in the role of a leader and facilitator and recalling the legal issues relating to physicians orders will assist in answering the question. Review the responsibilities of the nurse manager if you had difficulty with this question.

Level of Cognitive Ability: Comprehension
Client Needs: Safe and Effective Care Environment
Integrated Process: Nursing Process/Implementation
Content Area: Management of Care

Reference

Potter P, Perry A: *Fundamentals of nursing,* ed 6, St Louis, 2005, Mosby, p 797.

Figure/Illustration with a Fill-in-the-Blank

44. The nurse hangs a 1000 mL intravenous (IV) solution of D_5W (5% dextrose in water) at 9 AM and sets the infusion controller device to administer 100 mL/hr. On assessment of the IV infusion, the nurse expects that the safe amount of solution remaining in the IV bag at 2 PM will be represented at which level? (Refer to figure.)

Answer: _____

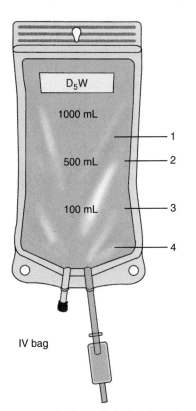

IV bag

From Kee J, Marshall S: *Clinical calculations: with applications to general and specialty areas,* ed 5, Philadelphia, 2004, Saunders.

Answer: 2

Rationale: The nurse hangs an IV solution at 9 AM and sets the IV solution to infuse at 100 mL/hr. At 2 PM, 5 hours later, the nurse would expect 500 mL of solution to be safely infused.

Test-Taking Strategy: Focus on the information in the question. Use simple mathematics to calculate that in a 5-hour period, 500 mL of fluid will infuse for a solution infusing at 100 mL/hr. Review flow rate infusions if you had difficulty with this question.

Level of Cognitive Ability: Comprehension
Client Needs: Safe and Effective Care Environment
Integrated Process: Nursing Process/Implementation
Content Area: Safety and Infection Control

Reference
Kee J, Marshall S: *Clinical calculations: with applications to general and specialty areas,* ed 5, Philadelphia, 2004, Saunders, pp 201-202.

Multiple Response

45. A nurse manager is reviewing the principles of surgical asepsis with the nursing staff. The nurse manager tells the staff that it is unnecessary to use the principles of surgical asepsis in which situations? Select all that apply.

❑ **1** Removing a dressing
❑ **2** Reapplying sterile dressings
❑ **3** Inserting an intravenous (IV) line
❑ **4** Inserting a urinary (Foley) catheter
❑ **5** Suctioning the tracheobronchial airway
❑ **6** Caring for an immunosuppressive client

Answer: 1, 6

Rationale: Surgical asepsis involves the use of sterile technique. Some examples of procedures where surgical asepsis is necessary include inserting an IV or urinary catheter, suctioning the tracheobronchial airway, and reapplying sterile dressings. Medical asepsis, or clean technique, includes procedures to reduce and prevent the spread of microorganisms. Removing a dressing can be done by clean technique using clean gloves (although reapplying the dressing requires surgical asepsis). Caring for an immunosuppressive client requires medical asepsis techniques.

Test-Taking Strategy: Focus on the subject, surgical asepsis, and note the strategic word *unnecessary*. This word indicates a negative event query and asks you to select the option(s) that are not surgical asepsis techniques. Recalling the definitions of medical and surgical asepsis will assist in answering this question. Review the difference between medical and surgical asepsis if you had difficulty with this question.

Level of Cognitive Ability: Application
Client Needs: Safe and Effective Care Environment
Integrated Process: Nursing Process/Implementation
Content Area: Safety and Infection Control

Reference
Potter P, Perry A: *Fundamentals of nursing*, ed 6, St Louis, 2005, Mosby, pp 788, 802.

REFERENCES

Black J, Hawks J: *Medical-surgical nursing: clinical management for positive outcomes,* ed 7, Philadelphia, 2005, Saunders.

Cohen E, Cesta T: *Nursing case management: from essentials to advanced practice applications,* ed 4, St Louis, 2005, Mosby.

Harkreader H, Hogan MA: *Fundamentals of nursing: caring and clinical judgment,* ed 2, Philadelphia, 2004, Saunders.

Huber D: *Leadership and nursing care management,* ed 3, Philadelphia, 2006, Saunders.

Ignatavicius D, Workman M: *Medical surgical nursing: critical thinking for collaborative care,* ed 5, Philadelphia, 2006, Saunders.

Kee J, Marshall S: *Clinical calculations: with applications to general and specialty areas,* ed 5, Philadelphia, 2004, Saunders.

Maurer F, Smith C: *Community public health nursing practice: health for families and populations,* ed 3, Philadelphia, 2005, Saunders.

National Council of State Boards of Nursing: www.ncsbn.org.

National Council of State Boards of Nursing: *National Council of State Boards of Nursing test plan for the NCLEX-RN® Examination* (effective date: April 2007), Chicago, 2006, The Council.

Perry A, Potter P: *Clinical nursing skills and techniques,* ed 6, St Louis, 2006, Mosby.

Potter P, Perry A: *Fundamentals of nursing,* ed 6, St Louis, 2005, Mosby.

CHAPTER **3**
▲▲▲

Health Promotion and Maintenance Questions

According to the National Council of State Boards of Nursing (NCSBN), the Health Promotion and Maintenance category makes up 6% to 12% of the examination questions (Box 3-1). This Client Needs category addresses the principles related to growth and development. This category also tests the nurse's knowledge, skills, and abilities required to assist the client, family members, and significant others in preventing health problems, recognizing early signs of alterations in health, and developing health practices that promote and support wellness. Some of the content related to this Client Needs category is identified in Box 3-2. Also refer to the *National Council of State Boards of Nursing Test Plan for the NCLEX-RN® Examination* (2006) on the NCSBN website at www.ncsbn.org for additional information.

The following section provides practice questions that address content related to the Client Needs category of Health Promotion and Maintenance. Although the NCSBN does not identify subcategories in this Client Needs category, the content areas for each question in this chapter are coded as either *Growth and Transitions Across the Life Span* or *Prevention and Detection of Health Alterations*.

BOX 3-1 ▲ HEALTH PROMOTION AND MAINTENANCE

Health Promotion and Maintenance = 6% to 12% of the questions

BOX 3-2 ▲ HEALTH PROMOTION AND MAINTENANCE CONTENT

- Encouraging adherence to immunization schedules
- Encouraging appropriate lifestyle choices
- Identifying expected growth and development milestones, developmental stages and transitions, and the changes that occur with the aging process
- Identifying high-risk behaviors
- Incorporating family planning, family systems, and human sexuality in the care of clients
- Incorporating the principles of teaching and learning
- Initiating measures to prevent disease
- Promoting health and wellness, health screening, and the use of health promotion programs
- Promoting self-care
- Providing maternity (antepartum, intrapartum, postpartum) and newborn care
- Recognizing expected body image changes
- Using physical assessment techniques

PRACTICE QUESTIONS

Multiple Response

46. Which factors increase the risk for hypothermia in an older client? Select all that apply.

❑ **1** Burns
❑ **2** Anemia
❑ **3** Hypoglycemia
❑ **4** Alcohol abuse
❑ **5** Hyperthyroidism
❑ **6** Ability to sense cold temperatures

Answer: 1, 2, 3, 4

Rationale: The median oral temperature of an older client is 96.8° F (36° C). Environmental temperatures below 65° F (18° C) may cause a serious drop in core body temperature to 95° F (35° C) or less in the older client. Numerous factors increase the risk of hypothermia in the older client, including thermoregulatory impairment (failure to sense cold); conditions that decrease heat production such as hypothyroidism, hypoglycemia, or anemia; conditions that increase heat loss (e.g., burns); or medications or substances that interfere with thermoregulation such as alcohol.

Test-Taking Strategy: Focus on the subject, the risks associated with hypothermia. Recall that hypothermia is an abnormally dangerous and low body temperature. Next think about the pathophysiology or effects of each item in the options to answer correctly. Review the risk factors for hypothermia in an older client if you had difficulty with this question.

Level of Cognitive Ability: Analysis
Client Needs: Health Promotion and Maintenance
Integrated Process: Nursing Process/Analysis
Content Area: Growth and Transitions Across the Life Span

Reference
Ebersole P, Hess P, Touhy T, et al: *Gerontological nursing and healthy aging,* ed 2, St Louis, 2005, Mosby, pp 452-453.

Multiple Response

47. A nurse caring for a client in labor plans to assess the fetal heart rate (FHR) at which specific times? Select all that apply.

❏ **1** Before voiding
❏ **2** Before ambulation
❏ **3** After vaginal examination
❏ **4** After rupture of the membranes
❏ **5** Before turning the client on her side
❏ **6** Before the administration of oxytocin (Pitocin)

Answer: 2, 3, 4, 6

Rationale: Assessment of the mother and fetus is continuous during the dynamic process of labor. However, for all clients the FHR needs to be assessed immediately after rupture of the membranes, vaginal examinations, or any other invasive procedure; before ambulation; and before the administration of oxytocin, since these activities or situations can cause alterations in the FHR. The FHR is also assessed in between contractions, during the contraction, and for at least 30 seconds after the contraction. It is not necessary to assess the FHR before voiding or turning the client to her side.

Test-Taking Strategy: Note that the subject of the question relates to the times at which FHR monitoring is necessary. Read each option and think about the effect that the activity or situation has on the FHR. Eliminate options 1 (before voiding) and 5 (before turning the client on her side) because these activities will not affect the FHR. Review care of the client in labor if you had difficulty with this question.

Level of Cognitive Ability: Application
Client Needs: Health Promotion and Maintenance
Integrated Process: Nursing Process/Planning
Content Area: Prevention and Detection of Health Alterations

Reference
Murray S, McKinney E: *Foundations of maternal-newborn nursing,* ed 4, Philadelphia, 2006, Saunders, p 328.

Multiple Response

48. A mother of a 3-year-old child asks the nurse what personal and social developmental milestones she can expect to see in her child. The nurse tells the mother to expect which of the following? Select all that apply.

- ❏ **1** Begins problem solving
- ❏ **2** Exhibits sexual curiosity
- ❏ **3** May begin to masturbate
- ❏ **4** Notices gender differences
- ❏ **5** Develops a sense of initiative
- ❏ **6** Develops positive self-esteem through skill acquisition and task completion

Answer: 2, 3, 4

Rationale: Personal and social developmental milestones of the 3-year-old include putting on articles of clothing; brushing teeth with help; washing and drying hands using soap and water; noticing gender differences and identifying with children of own gender; exhibiting sexual curiosity and possibly beginning to masturbate; knowing own name; and understanding the need to take turns and share, but perhaps not being ready to do so. Developmental milestones for the 4- and 5-year-old child include developing a sense of initiative and beginning to problem solve. Developing positive self-esteem through skill acquisition and task completion is characteristic of a 6- to 8-year-old child.

Test-Taking Strategy: Focus on the subject, the developmental milestones of a 3-year-old. Read each option carefully, thinking about what can be expected of a child at this age. This will assist in eliminating options 1, 5, and 6 because they are higher level abilities. Review the developmental milestones of a 3-year-old child if you had difficulty with this question.

Level of Cognitive Ability: Application
Client Needs: Health Promotion and Maintenance
Integrated Process: Teaching and Learning
Content Area: Growth and Transitions Across the Life Span

Reference
McKinney E, James S, Murray S, et al: *Maternal-child nursing,* ed 2, Philadelphia, 2005, Saunders, pp 120, 126, 136.

Multiple Response

49. A nurse at a community health care clinic is teaching parents about measures to take to prevent and manage obesity in children. The nurse determines that a parent needs additional teaching about these measures if the parent states she will do which of the following? Select all that apply.

- ❑ **1** Use foods as a reward.
- ❑ **2** Offer healthy foods options.
- ❑ **3** Avoid eating at fast-food restaurants.
- ❑ **4** Keep unhealthy food out of the house.
- ❑ **5** Allow eating in between meals and snack times.
- ❑ **6** Establish consistent times for meals and snacks.

Answer: 1, 5

Rationale: Parents can implement several measures to prevent and manage obesity in their children. These measures include not using food as a reward; establishing consistent times for meals and snacks, and not allowing eating in between; offering only healthy foods options; keeping unhealthy food out of the house; minimizing trips to fast-food restaurants; acting as a role model for children; encouraging the child to do fun, physical activities with the family; and praising the child for making appropriate food choices and for increasing physical activity levels.

Test-Taking Strategy: Note the strategic words *needs additional teaching*. These words indicate a negative event query and ask you to select the option(s) that are incorrect statements. Read each option and think about its effect on preventing and managing obesity; this will direct you to the correct options. Review these measures if you had difficulty with this question.

Level of Cognitive Ability: Analysis
Client Needs: Health Promotion and Maintenance
Integrated Process: Teaching and Learning
Content Area: Prevention and Detection of Health Alterations

Reference
McKinney E, James S, Murray S, et al: *Maternal-child nursing,* ed 2, Philadelphia, 2005, Saunders, p 144.

Figure/Illustration with a Fill-in-the-Blank

50. The nurse is percussing the anterior thorax and the abdomen for tones and expects to note dullness in which anatomical location? (Refer to figure.)

Answer: _____

Answer: 3

Rationale: Percussion involves tapping the body with the fingertips to set the underlying structures in motion and thus produce a sound. Dullness will be noted over the liver, located in the upper right quadrant of the abdomen and beneath the lower ribs on the right side. Tympany is the most common percussion tone heard in the abdomen and is due to the presence of gas. Resonance is the percussion tone heard between the ribs.

Test-Taking Strategy: Focus on the subject, the anatomical location in which dullness would be percussed. Recalling that dullness on percussion indicates the presence of an organ will assist in answering the question. Also recall that the presence of a mass would produce dullness on percussion and would be an abnormal finding. Review the technique of percussion and the expected findings if you had difficulty with this question.

Level of Cognitive Ability: Analysis
Client Needs: Health Promotion and Maintenance
Integrated Process: Nursing Process/Assessment
Content Area: Prevention and Detection of Health Alterations

Reference
Wilson S, Giddens J: *Health assessment for nursing practice,* ed 3, St Louis, 2005, Mosby, pp 344-345, 445-446.

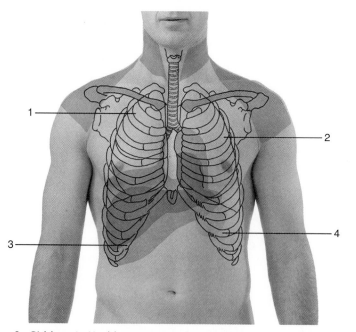

From Wilson S, Giddens J: *Health assessment for nursing practice,* ed 3, St Louis, 2005, Mosby.

Chart/Exhibit with a Fill-in-the-Blank

51. A client at the family planning clinic requests a prescription for oral contraceptives. The nurse determines that oral contraceptives are contraindicated because of which item documented in the client's history and physical examination in the medical record?

Answer: _____

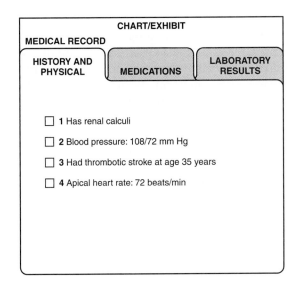

CHART/EXHIBIT

MEDICAL RECORD

| HISTORY AND PHYSICAL | MEDICATIONS | LABORATORY RESULTS |

☐ **1** Has renal calculi

☐ **2** Blood pressure: 108/72 mm Hg

☐ **3** Had thrombotic stroke at age 35 years

☐ **4** Apical heart rate: 72 beats/min

Answer: 3

Rationale: Oral contraceptives are contraindicated in women with a history of thrombophlebitis and thromboembolic disorders; cardiovascular or cerebrovascular diseases (including stroke); any estrogen-dependent cancer or breast cancer, or benign or malignant liver tumors; impaired liver function; hypertension; or diabetes mellitus with vascular involvement. Adverse effects of oral contraceptives include increased risk of superficial and deep venous thrombosis, pulmonary embolism, thrombotic stroke (or other types of strokes), myocardial infarction, and accelerations of preexisting breast tumors.

Test-Taking Strategy: Focus on the subject, the item that is a contraindication to the use of oral contraceptives. Eliminate items 2 and 4 because these are normal findings. To select from the remaining items, remember that oral contraceptives are contraindicated in cardiovascular or cerebrovascular disorders. Review contraindications to the use of oral contraceptives if you had difficulty with this question.

Level of Cognitive Ability: Analysis
Client Needs: Health Promotion and Maintenance
Integrated Process: Nursing Process/Analysis
Content Area: Prevention and Detection of Health Alterations

References
Kee J, Hayes E: *Pharmacology: a nursing process approach,* ed 5, St Louis, 2006, Mosby, p 846.
Murray S, McKinney E: *Foundations of maternal-newborn nursing,* ed 4, Philadelphia, 2006, Saunders, p 843.

Multiple Response

52. Identify the problems that adoptive parents may encounter. Select all that apply.

- ❑ **1** Set unrealistically high standard for themselves
- ❑ **2** Lack knowledge about the child's biological health history
- ❑ **3** Have difficulty assimilating if the child is adopted from another country
- ❑ **4** Have difficulty deciding when and how to tell the child about being adopted
- ❑ **5** Feel the need for more assistance and support in child-rearing than biological parents do
- ❑ **6** Face problems with child-rearing that are different from those encountered by natural parents

Answer: 1, 2, 3, 4

Rationale: Adoptive parents may add pressure to themselves by setting unrealistically high standards for themselves as parents. Additional problems adoptive families may face include possible lack of knowledge about the child's biological health history, difficulty assimilating if the child is adopted from another country, and difficulty deciding when and how to tell the child about being adopted. Otherwise, most problems faced by adoptive parents are no different from those encountered by natural parents. All parents want to be good parents. Both adoptive parents and biological parents need information, support, and guidance to prepare them to care for their child.

Test-Taking Strategy: Focus on the subject, problems that adoptive parents may encounter. Read each option and determine if the information distinctively relates to adoption. This will assist in answering the question. Review the problems faced by adoptive parents if you had difficulty with this question.

Level of Cognitive Ability: Analysis
Client Needs: Health Promotion and Maintenance
Integrated Process: Nursing Process/Analysis
Content Area: Growth and Transitions Across the Life Span

References
McKinney E, James S, Murray S, et al: *Maternal-child nursing,* ed 2, Philadelphia, 2005, Saunders, p 40.
Wong D, Perry S, Hockenberry M, et al: *Maternal child nursing care,* ed 3, St Louis, 2006, Mosby, p 905.

Multiple Response

53. A school nurse is performing screening examinations for scoliosis. The nurse assesses for which signs of scoliosis? Select all that apply.

❑ **1** Chest asymmetry
❑ **2** Equal waist angles
❑ **3** Unequal rib heights
❑ **4** Equal shoulder heights
❑ **5** Equal rib prominences
❑ **6** Lateral deviation and rotation of each vertebrae

Answer: 1, 3, 6

Rationale: Scoliosis is a lateral curvature of the spine. To ensure early detection and treatment, children ages 9 through 15 years should be screened for scoliosis; those at greatest risk are girls from 10 years of age through adolescence. The child should be unclothed or wearing only underpants so that the chest, back, and hips can be clearly seen. The child should stand with her or his weight equally on both feet, legs straight, and arms hanging loosely at the sides. The nurse then observes for the signs of scoliosis. These signs include nonpainful lateral curvature of the spine, a curve with one turn (C curve) or two compensating curves (S curve), lateral deviation and rotation of each vertebra, unequal shoulder heights, unequal waist angles, unequal rib prominences and chest asymmetry, and unequal rib heights.

Test-Taking Strategy: Focus on the subject, the signs of scoliosis, and recall the definition of scoliosis, a lateral curvature of the spine. Visualize this disorder and note the word *equal* in options 2, 4, and 5. This will assist in eliminating these options. Review the signs of scoliosis if you had difficulty with this question.

Level of Cognitive Ability: Application
Client Needs: Health Promotion and Maintenance
Integrated Process: Nursing Process/Assessment
Content Area: Prevention and Detection of Health Alterations

Reference
McKinney E, James S, Murray S, et al: *Maternal-child nursing*, ed 2, Philadelphia, 2005, Saunders, p 843.

Prioritizing (Ordered Response)

54. Identify in order of progression the gross motor development of an infant from ages 2 weeks to 15 months. (Number 1 is the first motor skill that develops at 2 weeks, and number 6 is the motor skill that develops at 15 months.)

___ Rolls over
___ Walks alone
___ Attempts to walk with support
___ Sits alone using hands for support
___ Raises the head and holds the position
___ Moves all extremities, kicking arms and legs when prone

Answer: 3, 6, 5, 4, 1, 2

Rationale: Between the ages of 2 weeks and 2 months the infant raises the head and holds the position. At age 2 months the infant moves all extremities, kicking the arms and legs when prone. By 3 to 6 months of age the infant rolls over. By 7 months of age the infant sits alone using the hands for support. By 12 months of age the infant attempts to walk with support or holds on to something stable. By 15 months of age the infant walks alone.

Test-Taking Strategy: Focus on the subject, the order of progression of the gross motor development of an infant. Read each option and visualize the progression of infant motor skills. This will assist in placing the skills in order. Review the gross motor development of an infant if you had difficulty with this question.

Level of Cognitive Ability: Analysis
Client Needs: Health Promotion and Maintenance
Integrated Process: Nursing Process/Assessment
Content Area: Growth and Transitions Across the Life Span

Reference
McKinney E, James S, Murray S, et al: *Maternal-child nursing,* ed 2, Philadelphia, 2005, Saunders, p 843.

Figure/Illustration with a Multiple Choice

55. The nurse reviews the results of a nonstress test performed on a pregnant client and interprets the finding as which of the following? (Refer to figure.)

❑ **1** Reactive
❑ **2** Abnormal
❑ **3** Nonreactive
❑ **4** Nonreassuring

Answer: 1

Rationale: A nonstress test assesses fetal well-being and evaluates the ability of the fetal heart to accelerate, often in association with fetal movement. Accelerations of the fetal heart rate are associated with adequate oxygenation, a healthy neural pathway, and the fetal heart's ability to respond to stimuli. A reactive test is described as at least two fetal heart rate accelerations, with or without fetal movement, occurring within a 20-minute period and peaking at least 15 beats/min above the baseline and lasting 15 seconds from baseline to baseline. This recording (see figure) identifies a reactive nonstress test. The fetal heart rate acceleration peaks at least 15 beats/min and lasts for at least 15 seconds in response to fetal movement. A nonreactive test is an abnormal or nonreassuring test. In a nonreactive test the recording does not demonstrate the required characteristics of a reactive test within a 40-minute period.

Test-Taking Strategy: Note the accelerations identified in the figure. Also note that options 2, 3, and 4 are comparable or alike in that they all indicate a nonreactive test result. Review interpretation of nonstress results if you had difficulty with this question.

Level of Cognitive Ability: Analysis
Client Needs: Health Promotion and Maintenance
Integrated Process: Nursing Process/Analysis
Content Area: Prevention and Detection of Health Alterations

Reference
McKinney E, James S, Murray S, et al: *Maternal-child nursing,* ed 2, Philadelphia, 2005, Saunders, p 332.

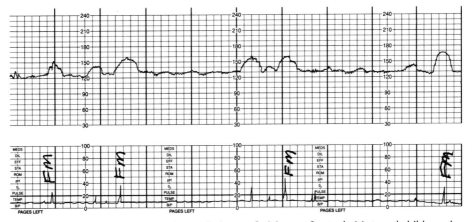

FM, Fetal movement. From McKinney E, James S, Murray S, et al: *Maternal-child nursing,* ed 2, Philadelphia, 2005, Saunders.

Multiple Response

56. Which of the following clients are at greatest risk for developing osteoporosis? Select all that apply.

   ❏ 1 An Asian woman
   ❏ 2 A large-boned, dark-skinned woman
   ❏ 3 A client who started menopause early
   ❏ 4 A client with a family history of the disease
   ❏ 5 A client who has a physically active lifestyle
   ❏ 6 A client with an inadequate intake of calcium and vitamin D

Answer: 1, 3, 4, 6

Rationale: Osteoporosis is a disorder characterized by abnormal loss of bone density and deterioration of bone tissue, with an increased fracture risk. Small-boned, fair-skinned, white and Asian women are at greatest risk for osteoporosis. Other risk factors include a family history of the disease, early menopause, and a sedentary lifestyle. Women who smoke, drink alcohol, or take corticosteroids or anticonvulsants, as well as those who consume excessive amounts of caffeine, also have increased risk for osteoporosis. Inadequate intake of calcium and vitamin D is a major risk factor because it results in abnormal loss of bone density and deterioration of bone tissue.

Test-Taking Strategy: Focus on the subject, the risk factors for osteoporosis. Recalling that osteoporosis is characterized by an abnormal loss of bone density and deterioration of bone tissue will assist in identifying the risk factors. Also remember that small-boned, fair-skinned, white and Asian women are at greatest risk for osteoporosis. Review these risk factors if you had difficulty with this question.

Level of Cognitive Ability: Analysis
Client Needs: Health Promotion and Maintenance
Integrated Process: Nursing Process/Assessment
Content Area: Prevention and Detection of Health Alterations

References
McKinney E, James S, Murray S, et al: *Maternal-child nursing*, ed 2, Philadelphia, 2005, Saunders, p 783.
Murray S, McKinney E: *Foundations of maternal-newborn nursing*, ed 4, Philadelphia, 2006, Saunders, p 904.

Multiple Response

57. A client is diagnosed with organic erectile dysfunction. The nurse explains to the client that which of the following are causes of this disorder? Select all that apply.

- ❑ **1** Stress
- ❑ **2** Depression
- ❑ **3** Vascular disease
- ❑ **4** Diabetes mellitus
- ❑ **5** Alcohol consumption
- ❑ **6** Use of antihypertensives

Answer: 3, 4, 5, 6

Rationale: Erectile dysfunction is the inability to achieve or maintain an erection for sexual intercourse. Organic erectile dysfunction is a gradual deterioration of function; the man first notices diminishing firmness and a decrease in frequency of erections. Causes include inflammation of the prostate, urethra, or seminal vesicles; surgical procedures such as prostatectomy; pelvic fractures or lumbosacral injuries; vascular diseases, including hypertension; chronic neurological conditions such as Parkinson's disease or multiple sclerosis; endocrine disorders such as diabetes mellitus or thyroid disorders; smoking and alcohol consumption; drugs; and poor overall health. Functional erectile dysfunction usually has a psychological cause.

Test-Taking Strategy: Focus on the subject, organic erectile dysfunction. Noting the strategic word *organic* and recalling that these types of disorders have a physiological cause will direct you to the correct options. Review the causes of organic erectile dysfunction if you had difficulty with this question.

Level of Cognitive Ability: Application
Client Needs: Health Promotion and Maintenance
Integrated Process: Teaching and Learning
Content Area: Growth and Transitions Across the Life Span

References

Ignatavicius D, Workman M: *Medical surgical nursing: critical thinking for collaborative care,* ed 5, Philadelphia, 2006, Saunders, p 1870.
Murray S, McKinney E: *Foundations of maternal-newborn nursing,* ed 4, Philadelphia, 2006, Saunders, p 858.

Multiple Response

58. Percussion is a physical assessment technique that is used to assess which of the following? Select all that apply.

❑ **1** Fluid in body cavities
❑ **2** Borders of body organs
❑ **3** Consistency of body organs
❑ **4** Mobility of organs and other structures
❑ **5** Resilience and resistance of tissue and organs
❑ **6** Location, size, and density of an underlying structure

Answer: 1, 2, 3, 6

Rationale: Percussion involves tapping the body with the fingertips to evaluate the size, borders, and consistency of body organs and to assess for fluid in body cavities. Through percussion, the location, size, and density of an underlying structure can be determined. Through palpation, assessment is done via the sense of touch. Measurements of specific physical signs, including resistance, resilience, roughness, texture, and mobility, can be made through palpation.

Test-Taking Strategy: Focus on the subject of the question, percussion, and recall that percussion involves tapping the body with the fingertips. Visualize the effect of this assessment technique to determine what it would evaluate. Review this assessment technique if you had difficulty with this question.

Level of Cognitive Ability: Analysis
Client Needs: Health Promotion and Maintenance
Integrated Process: Nursing Process/Assessment
Content Area: Prevention and Detection of Health Alterations

Reference
Potter P, Perry A: *Fundamentals of nursing*, ed 6, St Louis, 2005, Mosby, pp 675-676.

Prioritizing (Ordered Response)

59. A client arrives at the health care clinic complaining of a cough. List in order of priority the steps that the nurse takes to assess the client. (Number 1 is the first step and number 6 is the last step.)

____ Introduce self to the client.
____ Auscultate the thorax for breath sounds.
____ Inspect the anterior and posterior thorax.
____ Percuss the anterior and posterior thorax.
____ Palpate the anterior and posterior thorax.
____ Obtain data regarding complaints and personal and family history.

Answer: 1, 6, 3, 5, 4, 2

Rationale: The two components of health assessment are the history (collection of subjective data) and the physical examination (collection of objective data). The nurse always introduces himself or herself first to the client and explains the procedure for the assessment. The nurse next collects data regarding complaints and personal and family history and any other significant data. This is known as the interview and serves many useful purposes, including establishing a nurse-client relationship and identifying significant data that serve as a baseline for performing the physical assessment. The four basic techniques used in the physical examination are inspection, palpation, percussion, and auscultation, and they are generally performed in that order. Palpation follows inspection, except during examination of the abdomen, when palpation is done last so that it does not alter bowel sounds and change the findings on percussion and auscultation.

Test-Taking Strategy: To determine the order of priority, remember that the nurse always introduces himself or herself to the client on initial contact. Next recall the importance of establishing a nurse-client relationship. This assists in determining that obtaining data from the client is the next step. To determine the remaining orders of action, recall that physical assessment is performed in the following order: inspection, palpation, percussion, auscultation. Review physical assessment techniques if you had difficulty with this question.

Level of Cognitive Ability: Application
Client Needs: Health Promotion and Maintenance
Integrated Process: Nursing Process/Assessment
Content Area: Prevention and Detection of Health Alterations

Reference
Harkreader H, Hogan MA: *Fundamentals of nursing: caring and clinical judgment,* ed 2, Philadelphia, 2004, Saunders, pp 89, 92, 95, 129.

Multiple Response

60. The nurse provides information to a client about performing a breast-self examination (BSE). The nurse determines that the client needs additional information if the client makes which statements? Select all that apply.

❑ **1** "The BSE needs to be done monthly."

❑ **2** "Lumps in my armpit area are normal."

❑ **3** "I can palpate my breasts with soapy water while showering."

❑ **4** "I should perform the examination on the day that I start my period."

❑ **5** "When I squeeze my nipples, I should expect to note some discharge."

❑ **6** "I should stand before a mirror and inspect each breast for anything unusual."

Answer: 2, 4, 5

Rationale: The client is taught that BSE should be done once a month so that the client becomes familiar with the usual feel and appearance of the breasts. The examination is performed 2 or 3 days after menstruation ends, when the breasts are least likely to be tender and swollen. The client is taught to stand before a mirror and inspect each breast for anything unusual and to palpate each breast and axillary area. The client may perform this part of the examination in the shower using soap, which allows the fingers to glide easily over the skin. Any lumps (including lumps in the armpit) and nipple discharge are abnormal and need to be reported to the health care provider immediately.

Test-Taking Strategy: Note the strategic words *needs additional information*. These words indicate a negative event query and ask you to select the options that are incorrect statements. Read each option carefully, and remember that the examination is performed 2 or 3 days after menstruation ends, when the breasts are least likely to be tender and swollen. Also, recalling that any lumps (including lumps in the armpit) and nipple discharge are abnormal will assist in answering correctly. Review the procedure for BSE if you had difficulty with this question.

Level of Cognitive Ability: Analysis
Client Needs: Health Promotion and Maintenance
Integrated Process: Teaching and Learning
Content Area: Prevention and Detection of Health Alterations

Reference
Potter P, Perry A: *Fundamentals of nursing*, ed 6, St Louis, 2005, Mosby, p 736.

Multiple Response

61. A nurse employed in a well-baby clinic is preparing to administer the scheduled recommended immunizations to a 2-month-old infant. The nurse reviews the infant's immunization schedule and notes documentation that the infant received the first dose of hepatitis B (Hep B) vaccine at birth. After consultation with the pediatrician, the nurse should prepare to administer which vaccines at this time? Select all that apply.

- ❑ **1** Pneumococcal (PCV)
- ❑ **2** Inactivated poliovirus (IPV)
- ❑ **3** Hepatitis B (Hep B) (second dose)
- ❑ **4** *Haemophilus influenzae* type b conjugate (Hib)
- ❑ **5** Varicella; measles, mumps, and rubella (MMR)
- ❑ **6** Diphtheria and tetanus toxoids and acellular pertussis (DTaP)

Answer: 1, 2, 3, 4, 6

Rationale: All newborns need to receive the Hep B vaccine at birth, with the second dose administered at 1 to 2 months of age, and a third dose at or later than 24 weeks of age. DTaP is administered at 2, 4, and 6 months of age; the fourth dose is administered as early as age 12 months as long as 6 months have elapsed since the third dose. Hib is administered at ages 2 and 4 months with a final dose administered at age 12 months or older. IPV is administered at ages 2 and 4 months and then at age 4 to 6 years. MMR is administered at age 12 months with the second dose at age 4 to 6 years. Varicella vaccine is administered at age 12 months or older.

Test-Taking Strategy: Specific knowledge regarding the recommended childhood immunization schedule is needed to answer this question. Note that the infant is 2 months of age, and remember that a 2-month-old infant is scheduled for Hep B, DTaP, Hib, IPV, and PCV. Review the recommended childhood immunization schedule if you had difficulty with this question.

Level of Cognitive Ability: Application
Client Needs: Health Promotion and Maintenance
Integrated Process: Nursing Process/Implementation
Content Area: Prevention and Detection of Health Alterations

Reference
Department of Health and Human Services, Centers for Disease Control and Prevention: *Recommended childhood and adolescent immunization schedule: United States: 2006*, retrieved May 17, 2006, from www.vaccineplace.com/syndication/pdf/child-schedule.pdf.

Multiple Response

62. A community health nurse is providing an educational session on the early detection of testicular cancer and includes which of the following information? Select all that apply.

❑ **1** A testicular tumor is very painful.

❑ **2** Testicular self-examination (TSE)should be performed monthly.

❑ **3** The best time to perform a TSE is before taking a shower.

❑ **4** Lumps that are smaller than a pea felt when doing the TSE are normal.

❑ **5** Testicular cancer most commonly occurs in men between the ages of 15 and 35 years.

❑ **6** A dragging sensation or feeling of heaviness in the scrotum is a sign of a testicular tumor.

Answer: 2, 5, 6

Rationale: Testicular cancer is the most common and serious solid tumor cancer in men between the ages of 15 and 35 years. A dragging sensation or feeling of heaviness in the scrotum is a sign of a testicular tumor, and the tumor is painless. The client is taught to perform a monthly TSE and to immediately report the presence of any lump regardless of size to the health care provider. The best time to perform the TSE is after bathing because the warm water causes the scrotum to relax and makes the testicles easier to examine.

Test-Taking Strategy: Read each option carefully. Thinking about the procedure for performing and palpating the testicle during TSE will assist in eliminating the option that indicates performing TSE before taking a shower. Next, recalling that the presence of any lump needs to be reported will assist in eliminating the option that indicates lumps smaller than a pea are normal. To select from the remaining options, remember that testicular cancer most commonly occurs in men between the ages of 15 and 35 years and that an early sign is a painless dragging sensation, or feeling of heaviness in the scrotum.

Level of Cognitive Ability: Application
Client Needs: Health Promotion and Maintenance
Integrated Process: Teaching and Learning
Content Area: Prevention and Detection of Health Alterations

References
Black J, Hawks J: *Medical-surgical nursing: clinical management for positive outcomes,* ed 7, Philadelphia, 2005, Saunders, pp 1005, 1037.
Ignatavicius D, Workman M: *Medical surgical nursing: critical thinking for collaborative care,* ed 5, Philadelphia, 2006, Saunders, pp 1871-1872.

Multiple Response

63. A nurse teaches a client at risk for coronary artery disease about lifestyle changes needed to reduce his risks. The nurse determines that the client understands these necessary lifestyle changes if the client makes which statements? Select all that apply.

- ❏ **1** "I will cut down on my smoking habit."
- ❏ **2** "I will be sure to include some exercise such as walking in my daily activities."
- ❏ **3** "I will work at losing some weight so that my weight is at normal range for my age."
- ❏ **4** "I will limit my sodium intake every day and avoid eating high-sodium foods such as hot dogs."
- ❏ **5** "It is acceptable to eat red meat and cheese every day as I have been doing, as long as I cut down on the butter."
- ❏ **6** "I will schedule regular physician appointments for physical examinations and monitoring my blood pressure."

Answer: 2, 3, 4, 6

Rationale: Coronary artery disease affects the arteries that provide blood, oxygen, and nutrients to the myocardium. Modifiable risk factors include elevated serum cholesterol levels, cigarette smoking, hypertension, impaired glucose tolerance, obesity, physical inactivity, and stress. The client is instructed to stop smoking (not cut down), and the nurse should provide the client with resources to do so. The client is also instructed to maintain a normal weight, include physical activity in the daily schedule, and follow up with regular physician appointments for physical examinations and monitoring blood pressure. The client is also instructed to limit sodium intake and foods high in cholesterol, including red meat and cheese.

Test-Taking Strategy: Focus on the subject, lifestyle changes to reduce the risk of coronary artery disease. Think about the pathophysiology associated with coronary artery disease. Read each option carefully and recall that coronary artery disease affects the arteries that provide blood, oxygen, and nutrients to the myocardium. This will assist in selecting the correct options. Review the lifestyle changes to reduce the risk of coronary artery disease if you had difficulty with this question.

Level of Cognitive Ability: Analysis
Client Needs: Health Promotion and Maintenance
Integrated Process: Nursing Process/Evaluation
Content Area: Prevention and Detection of Health Alterations

Reference
Ignatavicius D, Workman M: *Medical surgical nursing: critical thinking for collaborative care,* ed 5, Philadelphia, 2006, Saunders, pp 842-844.

Multiple Response

64. Identify the factors that the nurse should consider for teaching a child about his or her disease and related health care measures. Select all that apply.

    ❑ 1 A child rarely forms misconceptions.
    ❑ 2 The older the child, the shorter the attention span.
    ❑ 3 A child's imagination may create greater fear than the truth.
    ❑ 4 A child may regress developmentally in a situation of illness.
    ❑ 5 It is not necessary to assess the child's knowledge before teaching.
    ❑ 6 A child may better manage uncomfortable information through role-playing.

Answer: 3, 4, 6

Rationale: For children, the teaching-learning process may be fundamentally different than that used for adults, and the nurse needs to adjust the complexity and volume of information based on the child's age and cognitive level. The factors that need to be addressed when teaching children include the following: trust is essential to a therapeutic relationship; in general, the younger the child, the shorter the attention span; assessing the child's knowledge is important because children are exposed to various levels of information about health care; children form misconceptions easily, and a child's imagination may create greater fear than the truth; a child may regress developmentally in a situation of illness; and a child may better manage uncomfortable information through role-playing.

Test-Taking Strategy: Focus on the subject, factors to consider for teaching a child. Read each option carefully and think about the concepts of growth and development. This will assist in selecting the correct options. Review these factors if you had difficulty with this question.

Level of Cognitive Ability: Application
Client Needs: Health Promotion and Maintenance
Integrated Process: Teaching and Learning
Content Area: Growth and Transitions Across the Life Span

Reference
Harkreader H, Hogan MA: *Fundamentals of nursing: caring and clinical judgment,* ed 2, Philadelphia, 2004, Saunders, p 263.

Multiple Response

65. A community health nurse is providing information about the risks of cervical cancer to a women's health group. The nurse explains that which of the following are risk factors for this type of cancer? Select all that apply.

- ❑ **1** Multiparity
- ❑ **2** White race
- ❑ **3** Multiple sex partners
- ❑ **4** Infection with herpes simplex virus (HSV)
- ❑ **5** An age of more than 18 years at first intercourse
- ❑ **6** Intrauterine exposure to diethylstilbestrol (DES)

Answer: 1, 3, 4, 6

Rationale: Cervical cancer is a progression from totally normal cervical cells to premalignant changes in appearance of cervical cells (dysplasia), to changes in function and, ultimately, transformation to cancer. The exact cause of cervical cancer is unknown, but many risk factors are involved. These risk factors include African-American race; Native American Indian race; multiparity; an age of less than 18 years at first intercourse; an age of less than 18 years at first pregnancy; multiple sex partners; smoking; infection with HSV; infection with cytomegalovirus; human immunodeficiency virus and acquired immunodeficiency syndrome; low socioeconomic status; sexual partner who had a previous partner who developed cervical cancer; and intrauterine exposure to DES.

Test-Taking Strategy: Specific knowledge regarding the risk factors associated with cervical cancer is needed to answer this question. Therefore the best way to answer questions correctly that address cervical risk factors is to learn what these risk factors are. Cervical cancer is an important content area, so review these risk factors if you had difficulty with this question.

Level of Cognitive Ability: Application
Client Needs: Health Promotion and Maintenance
Integrated Process: Teaching and Learning
Content Area: Prevention and Detection of Health Alterations

Reference
Ignatavicius D, Workman M: *Medical surgical nursing: critical thinking for collaborative care,* ed 5, Philadelphia, 2006, p 1843.

REFERENCES

Black J, Hawks J: *Medical-surgical nursing: clinical management for positive outcomes,* ed 7, Philadelphia, 2005, Saunders.

Department of Health and Human Services, Centers for Disease Control and Prevention: *Recommended childhood and adolescent immunization schedule: United States: 2006,* retrieved May 17, 2006, from www.vaccineplace.com/syndication/pdf/child-schedule.pdf.

Ebersole P, Hess P, Touhy T, et al: *Gerontological nursing and healthy aging,* ed 2, St Louis, 2005, Mosby.

Harkreader H, Hogan MA: *Fundamentals of nursing: caring and clinical judgment,* ed 2, Philadelphia, 2004, Saunders.

Ignatavicius D, Workman M: *Medical surgical nursing: critical thinking for collaborative care,* ed 5, Philadelphia, 2006, Saunders.

Kee J, Hayes E: *Pharmacology: a nursing process approach,* ed 5, St Louis, 2006, Mosby.

McKinney E, James S, Murray S, et al: *Maternal-child nursing,* ed 2, Philadelphia, 2005, Saunders.

Murray S, McKinney E: *Foundations of maternal-newborn nursing,* ed 4, Philadelphia, 2006.

National Council of State Boards of Nursing: www.ncsbn.org.

National Council of State Boards of Nursing: *National Council of State Boards of Nursing test plan for the NCLEX-RN® Examination* (effective date: April 2007), Chicago, 2006, The Council.

Potter P, Perry A: *Fundamentals of nursing,* ed 6, St Louis, 2005, Mosby.

Wilson S, Giddens J: *Health assessment for nursing practice,* ed 3, St Louis, 2005, Mosby.

Wong D, Perry S, Hockenberry M, et al: *Maternal child nursing care,* ed 3, St Louis, 2006, Mosby.

CHAPTER 4

Psychosocial Integrity Questions

According to the National Council of State Boards of Nursing (NCSBN), the Psychosocial Integrity category makes up 6% to 12% of the examination questions (Box 4-1). This Client Needs category addresses the nurse's knowledge, skill, and abilities required to promote and support the client, family, and significant others' ability to cope, adapt, and problem solve during stressful events. This Client Needs category also addresses the emotional, mental, and social well-being of the client, family, and significant other, and the knowledge, skill, and ability required to care for the client with an acute or chronic mental illness. Some of the content related to this Client Needs category is identified in Box 4-2. Also refer to the *National Council of State Boards of Nursing Test Plan for the NCLEX-RN® Examination* (2006) on the NCSBN website at www.ncsbn.org for additional information.

The following section provides practice questions that address content related to the Client Needs category Psychosocial Integrity. Although the NCSBN does not identify subcategories in this Client Needs category, the content areas for each question in this chapter is coded as either *Psychosocial Adaptation* or *Mental Health Disorders*.

BOX 4-1 ▲ PSYCHOSOCIAL INTEGRITY

Psychosocial Integrity = 6% to 12% of the questions

BOX 4-2 ▲ PSYCHOSOCIAL INTEGRITY CONTENT

- Addressing cultural diversity issues in caring for the client
- Assessing family dynamics
- Assessing for abuse or neglect
- Assessing the client's support systems
- Assisting the client to use coping mechanisms
- Caring for the client with a chemical or other dependency
- Considering end-of-life and grief and loss issues
- Considering religious and spiritual influences on health
- Discussing situational role changes and unexpected body image changes with the client
- Implementing behavioral interventions as indicated
- Implementing crisis intervention measures
- Monitoring for sensory and perceptual alterations
- Providing stress management techniques
- Providing a therapeutic environment
- Using mental health concepts as a guide in caring for the client
- Using therapeutic communication techniques

PRACTICE QUESTIONS

Multiple Response

66. A battered woman seen in the emergency department requires tertiary intervention because of repeated abuse. Which nursing interventions are appropriate? Select all that apply.

❑ 1 Report the abuse to the police.
❑ 2 Provide medications to relieve pain and anxiety.
❑ 3 Explore family and friends as support possibilities.
❑ 4 Focus on the woman's strengths, endurance, and abilities.
❑ 5 Avoid discussing the implications of pressing charges against the batterer.
❑ 6 Discourage the woman from discussing the events leading to past and present abuse situations.

Answer: 1, 2, 3, 4

Rationale: Tertiary prevention is necessary when a woman has been repeatedly abused. The focus is on helping the abused woman to overcome the physical and psychological effects of the abuse and on preventing future abuse. Some of the interventions include reporting the abuse to the police to provide for safety; providing medications to relieve pain and anxiety; exploring family and friends as support possibilities to increase the woman's awareness of potential support; focusing on the woman's strengths, endurance, and abilities to increase her self-esteem; discussing the implications of pressing charges against the batterer to increase her awareness of abuse implications; and encouraging the woman to discuss the events leading to past and present abuse situations (this helps to reduce guilt and shame).

Test-Taking Strategy: Focus on the subject of the question, tertiary intervention for abuse. Recall that the focus of tertiary prevention is on helping the abused woman overcome the physical and psychological effects of the abuse and on preventing future abuse. Next read and visualize each intervention and relate it to the focus of tertiary intervention to select correctly. Review tertiary interventions for the battered woman if you had difficulty with this question.

Level of Cognitive Ability: Application
Client Needs: Psychosocial Integrity
Integrated Process: Nursing Process/Implementation
Content Area: Psychosocial Adaptation

Reference
Fortinash K, Holoday-Worret P: *Psychiatric mental health nursing,* ed 3, St Louis, 2004, Mosby, pp 528-529.

Multiple Response

67. The nurse is caring for a client who is a survivor of an external disaster. The client begins to display behaviors not demonstrated before. Which of the following manifestations would indicate to the nurse that the client may be experiencing posttraumatic stress disorder (PTSD)? Select all that apply.

- ❏ **1** Irritability and sleep disturbances
- ❏ **2** Flashbacks or recollections of the disaster
- ❏ **3** Regression to an earlier developmental stage
- ❏ **4** A feeling of estrangement or detachment from others
- ❏ **5** Consistent discussion and rationalizing as to why the disaster occurred
- ❏ **6** Repression or the inability to remember an important aspect associated with the disaster

Answer: 1, 2, 4, 6

Rationale: PTSD is characterized by a sustained maladaptive response to a traumatic event. In this condition the client experiences recurrent and intrusive recollections of the event (flashbacks), has recurrent dreams of the event, acts or feels as though the event were recurring, and experiences psychological distress when internal or external cues resemble the event. The individual avoids stimuli associated with the trauma or event (thoughts, feelings, conversations about the event, and persons or places that evoke memories of the event). The individual also is unable to remember an important aspect of the event (repression) and experiences somatic symptoms such as irritability and sleep disturbances. Regression to an earlier developmental stage and consistent discussion and rationalizing as to why the disaster occurred are not characteristics of PTSD.

Test-Taking Strategy: Focus on the client's diagnosis and recall that PTSD is a condition characterized by a sustained maladaptive response to a traumatic event. Read each option and associate the manifestation with the description of the disorder to answer correctly. Review manifestations indicative of PTSD if you had difficulty with this question.

Level of Cognitive Ability: Analysis
Client Needs: Psychosocial Integrity
Integrated Process: Nursing Process/Assessment
Content Area: Mental Health Disorders

References
Fortinash K, Holoday-Worret P: *Psychiatric mental health nursing,* ed 3, St Louis, 2004, Mosby, p 180.
Mosby's medical, nursing, and allied health dictionary, ed 7, St Louis, 2006, Mosby, p 1504.

Multiple Response

68. The nurse is performing an assessment of an adolescent client who has experienced family violence in the home. Which behavioral symptoms in the adolescent are likely to occur as a long-term effect of the family violence? Select all that apply.

- ❏ **1** Failing grades
- ❏ **2** Violent behaviors
- ❏ **3** Increased self-esteem
- ❏ **4** Running away from home
- ❏ **5** Difficulty forming relationships
- ❏ **6** Increased incidence of theft and police arrests

Answer: 1, 2, 4, 5, 6

Rationale: A violent family is one in which at least one family member is using physical or sexual force against another that results in physically or emotionally destructive injury or both. Behavioral symptoms that most likely occur in the adolescent as long-term effects of the family violence include failing grades; difficulty forming relationships; increased incidence of theft, police arrest, and violent behaviors; seductive or promiscuous behaviors; and running away from home. Poor self-esteem is likely to occur.

Test-Taking Strategy: Focus on the subject, the behavioral symptoms in the adolescent that are likely to occur as a long-term effect of family violence. Read each option and think about the description of family violence to assist in answering correctly. Remember that poor self-esteem is likely to occur. Review these behavioral symptoms if you had difficulty with this question.

Level of Cognitive Ability: Analysis
Client Needs: Psychosocial Integrity
Integrated Process: Nursing Process/Assessment
Content Area: Psychosocial Adaptation

Reference
Varcarolis E, Carson V, Shoemaker N: *Foundations of psychiatric mental health nursing,* ed 5, Philadelphia, 2006, Saunders, pp 506-507.

Multiple Response

69. The emergency department nurse implements which measures for a client experiencing a severe level of anxiety? Select all that apply.

- ❏ **1** Remain with the client.
- ❏ **2** Place the client in seclusion.
- ❏ **3** Place the client in a quiet room.
- ❏ **4** Minimize environmental stimuli.
- ❏ **5** Use clear and simple statements and repeat statements.
- ❏ **6** Use primarily dramatic nonverbal language to attract the client's attention.

Answer: 1, 3, 4, 5

Rationale: A client experiencing a severe level of anxiety is unable to solve problems and may have a poor grasp of what is happening in the environment. The nurse should remain with the client, maintain a calm manner, minimize environmental stimuli, and move the client to a quiet setting. Since the person with severe anxiety has difficulty concentrating and processing information, the nurse should use clear and simple statements and repetition and a low-pitched voice, speaking slowly. Dramatic nonverbal language will increase anxiety. The nurse should assess the person's need for medication or seclusion, but these interventions are considered only after other interventions have been tried and have not been successful.

Test-Taking Strategy: Focus on the subject, a client experiencing a severe level of anxiety. Visualize each intervention. Recall that seclusion is considered only after other interventions have been tried and failed and that dramatic nonverbal language will increase anxiety. Review the interventions for a client with severe anxiety if you had difficulty with this question.

Level of Cognitive Ability: Application
Client Needs: Psychosocial Integrity
Integrated Process: Nursing Process/Implementation
Content Area: Mental Health Disorders

Reference
Varcarolis E, Carson V, Shoemaker N: *Foundations of psychiatric mental health nursing*, ed 5, Philadelphia, 2006, Saunders, p 216.

Figure/Illustration with a Fill-in-the-Blank

70. A client with a diagnosis of schizophrenia is experiencing visual hallucinations. The nurse determines that this symptom is related to an alteration in brain function in which lobe of the cerebrum? (Refer to figure.)

Answer: _____

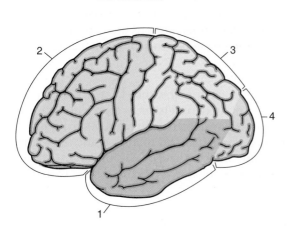

From Fortinash K, Holoday-Worret P: *Psychiatric mental health nursing*, ed 3, St Louis, 2004, Mosby.

Answer: 4

Rationale: The occipital lobe of the cerebrum (option 4) is located in the back of the head and is primarily responsible for seeing and receiving information via the eyes. Visual hallucinations indicate an alteration in brain function in this lobe. The temporal lobe (option 1) lies beneath the skull on both sides of the brain and is primarily responsible for hearing and receiving information via the ears. Symptoms indicating an alteration of function in the temporal lobe include auditory hallucinations, sensory aphasia, alterations in memory, and altered emotional responses. The frontal lobe (option 2) is located in the anterior or front area of the brain and is primarily responsible for motor functions, higher thought processes such as decision making, intellectual insight and judgment, and expression of emotion. Symptoms indicating an alteration of function in the frontal lobe include changes in affect, alteration in language production, alteration in motor function, impulsive behavior, and impaired decision making. The parietal lobe lies beneath the skull (option 3) and is primarily responsible for association and sensory perception. Symptoms indicating an alteration of function in the parietal lobe include alterations in sensory perceptions, difficulty with time concepts and calculating numbers, alteration in personal hygiene, and poor attention span.

Test-Taking Strategy: Focus on the strategic words *visual hallucinations*. Use concepts related to anatomy and physiology of the brain to answer this question. Recalling the location of the occipital lobe and that this lobe is primarily responsible for seeing and receiving information via the eyes will assist in answering correctly. Review the lobes of the cerebrum and the symptoms of dysfunction if you had difficulty with this question.

Level of Cognitive Ability: Analysis
Client Needs: Psychosocial Integrity
Integrated Process: Nursing Process/Assessment
Content Area: Mental Health Disorders

Reference
Fortinash K, Holoday-Worret P: *Psychiatric mental health nursing*, ed 3, St Louis, 2004, Mosby, pp 35-36.

Multiple Response

71. A nurse is interviewing the wife of a client who is a substance abuser. The nurse assesses the wife for which of the following behaviors that are indicative of codependence? Select all that apply.

- ❏ **1** States that she hides her husband's alcohol supply
- ❏ **2** States that she feels guilty about her husband's behavior
- ❏ **3** States that she doesn't spend time thinking about her husband
- ❏ **4** States that she finds excuses for her husband's substance abuse
- ❏ **5** States that she expects her husband to take care of his own legal or financial problems
- ❏ **6** States that she avoids social functions because of concern or shame about her husband's behavior

Answer: 1, 2, 4, 6

Rationale: People who are codependent often exhibit over-responsible behavior, doing for others what others could just as well do for themselves. A codependent person has a constellation of maladaptive thoughts, feelings, behaviors, and attitudes that effectively prevent him or her from living a full and satisfying life. Some of these behaviors include attempting to control someone else's substance use; spending inordinate time thinking about the substance abuser; finding excuses for the substance abuser; covering up for the substance abuser's problem or lying; avoiding family and social functions because of concern or shame about the substance abuser's behavior; making threats about the substance abuser's problem and failing to follow through; searching for, hiding, and destroying the substance abuser's alcohol supply; feeling guilty about the substance abuser's behavior; and bailing the substance abuser out of legal or financial problems.

Test-Taking Strategy: Focus on the subject, behaviors that are indicative of codependence. As you read each option, think about the description of a codependent person and recall that people who are codependent often exhibit overresponsible behavior, doing for others what others could just as well do for themselves. This will assist in identifying the correct answers. Review the behaviors of a codependent person if you had difficulty with this question.

Level of Cognitive Ability: Analysis
Client Needs: Psychosocial Integrity
Integrated Process: Nursing Process/Assessment
Content Area: Psychosocial Adaptation

Reference

Varcarolis E, Carson V, Shoemaker N: *Foundations of psychiatric mental health nursing,* ed 5, Philadelphia, 2006, Saunders, p 551.

Multiple Response

72. Which of the following would the nurse identify as a situational crisis? Select all that apply.

   ❑ 1 Divorce
   ❑ 2 Retirement
   ❑ 3 Loss of a job
   ❑ 4 An earthquake
   ❑ 5 The birth of a child
   ❑ 6 Death of a loved one

Answer: 1, 3, 6

Rationale: A situational crisis arises from an external rather than an internal source and often is unanticipated. Examples of external situations that can precipitate a situational crisis include the loss of a job, the death of a loved one, an abortion, a change in job, a change in financial status, divorce, and severe physical or mental illness. A maturational crisis occurs at a developmental stage; examples include marriage, the birth of a child, and retirement. An adventitious crisis, or crisis of disaster, is not a part of everyday life and is unplanned or accidental. This type of crisis can result from a natural disaster (flood, fire, earthquake), a national disaster (acts of terrorism, war, riots, airplane crashes), or a crime of violence (rape, assault, murder, bombing, spousal or child abuse).

Test-Taking Strategy: Focus on the subject, a situational crisis. Read each option and recall that a situational crisis arises from an external rather than an internal source and often is unanticipated. This will assist in selecting the correct answers. Review examples of situational crises if you had difficulty with this question.

Level of Cognitive Ability: Analysis
Client Needs: Psychosocial Integrity
Integrated Process: Nursing Process/Assessment
Content Area: Psychosocial Adaptation

Reference
Varcarolis E, Carson V, Shoemaker N: *Foundations of psychiatric mental health nursing,* ed 5, Philadelphia, 2006, Saunders, pp 458-459.

Multiple Response

73. A pregnant client, suspected of being physically abused by her husband, is brought to the emergency department after being found bleeding from her head by a neighbor. In evaluating the crisis situation, which questions should the nurse specifically ask to assess the client's perception of the precipitating event? Select all that apply.

❏ **1** Where do you go to worship?
❏ **2** Who is available to help you?
❏ **3** How does this situation affect your life?
❏ **4** Describe how you are feeling right now.
❏ **5** To whom do you talk when you are upset?
❏ **6** How do you see this event as affecting your future?

Answer: 3, 4, 6

Rationale: In a crisis situation the nurse's initial task is to assess the individual or family and the problem. Assessing the client's perception of the precipitating event will assist in clearly defining the problem, which will result in identifying a more effective solution. Examples of some questions that the nurse can ask to assess the client's perception of the precipitating event include: Has anything particularly upsetting happened to you within the past few days or weeks? What was happening in your life before you started to feel this way? What leads you to seek help now? Describe how you are feeling right now. How does this situation affect your life? How do you see this event as affecting your future? What would need to be done to resolve this situation? The other questions listed—Where do you go to worship? Who is available to help you? and To whom do you talk when you are upset?—assess situational supports, not the client's perception of the precipitating event.

Test-Taking Strategy: Focus on the strategic words *the client's perception of the precipitating event.* This will assist in determining the correct questions to ask the client. The incorrect answers assess situational supports, not the client's perception of the precipitating event. Review assessment of a client in crisis if you had difficulty with this question.

Level of Cognitive Ability: Analysis
Client Needs: Psychosocial Integrity
Integrated Process: Nursing Process/Assessment
Content Area: Psychosocial Adaptation

References
McKinney E, James S, Murray S, et al: *Maternal-child nursing,* ed 2, Philadelphia, 2005, Saunders, pp 610-613.
Varcarolis E, Carson V, Shoemaker N: *Foundations of psychiatric mental health nursing,* ed 5, Philadelphia, 2006, Saunders, p 460.

Multiple Response

74. A nurse is performing an assessment on a 34-year-old primigravida client who has been a marathon runner for several years. The client verbalizes concern because she is no longer able to run in marathons and is concerned about the brown discoloration on her face and her increasing size. Which statements by the nurse are therapeutic? Select all that apply.

   ❏ 1 "I can see you're disappointed at not being able to run."
   ❏ 2 "Tell me how you are feeling about the changes in your body."
   ❏ 3 "Don't worry. Your body will go back to normal after delivery."
   ❏ 4 "You need to ask your obstetrician about whether or not you can run."
   ❏ 5 "Wait and see. You will be back to marathon running after delivery before you know it."
   ❏ 6 "Some of the changes in pregnancy are permanent and that is the price that you have to pay for that bundle of joy."

Answer: 1, 2

Rationale: The client is concerned about the body changes and life changes being experienced as a result of pregnancy. Therapeutic communication techniques include focusing on the client's feelings and concerns and acknowledging these concerns by the techniques of clarifying (option 1) and encouraging discussion of feelings (option 2). Telling a client "not to worry" (option 3), avoiding discussion of the client's feelings (options 5 and 6), and placing the client's feelings on hold (option 4) are nontherapeutic communication techniques.

Test-Taking Strategy: Read each statement carefully. Use of therapeutic communication techniques will assist in determining the correct nursing statements. Review these therapeutic communication techniques if you had difficulty with this question.

Level of Cognitive Ability: Application
Client Needs: Psychosocial Integrity
Integrated Process: Communication and Documentation
Content Area: Psychosocial Adaptation

References
McKinney E, James S, Murray S, et al: *Maternal-child nursing,* ed 2, Philadelphia, 2005, Saunders, pp 30-32, 257, 282-283.
Murray S, McKinney E: *Foundations of maternal-newborn nursing,* ed 4, Philadelphia, 2006, Saunders, p 153.

Multiple Response

75. The nurse is performing a socioeconomic assessment of a Chinese client. Which questions would be appropriate for the nurse to ask? Select all that apply.

   ❑ 1 "What do you do for a living?"
   ❑ 2 "How much money do you make yearly?"
   ❑ 3 "Do you have a primary health care provider?"
   ❑ 4 "How many years of school did you complete?"
   ❑ 5 "How different is your life here from in your homeland?"
   ❑ 6 "What type of work did you do back in your homeland?"

Answer: 1, 3, 4, 5, 6

Rationale: Cultural assessment is a systematic and comprehensive examination of the cultural care values, beliefs, and practices of individuals, families, and communities and is important to the total care of any client. Aspects to assess include biocultural history and socioeconomic status (distinct health risks can be attributed to the ecological and socioeconomic context of the culture) and the client's country of origin. Other aspects to assess include religious and spiritual beliefs (to determine major influences in the client's worldview about health and illness, pain and suffering, and life and death), communication patterns (which reflect core cultural values of a society), time orientation (this information can be useful in planning a day of care, setting up appointments for procedures, and helping a client plan self-care activities in the home), caring beliefs and practices (to identify the central values of a culture), and previous experiences with professional health care (which may have implications for adherence to therapies and continuing access of services). Some specific questions to ask when performing a socioeconomic assessment include: What do you do for a living? Do you have a primary health care provider? How many years of school did you complete? How different is your life here from in your homeland? and What type of work did you do back in your homeland? Asking the client about his or her yearly income is inappropriate, unnecessary, and unrelated to health care resources.

Test-Taking Strategy: Focus on the subject, a socioeconomic assessment. Read each assessment question and think about its effect with regard to health risks, health care, and health care resources. This will assist in determining the correct assessment questions. Review the components of a socioeconomic assessment if you had difficulty with this question.

Level of Cognitive Ability: Analysis
Client Needs: Psychosocial Integrity
Integrated Process: Nursing Process/Assessment
Content Area: Psychosocial Adaptation

Reference
Potter P, Perry A: *Fundamentals of nursing,* ed 6, St Louis, 2005, Mosby, pp 131-134.

Multiple Response

76. A nurse is caring for a client with end-stage renal disease. What areas are appropriate to assess to determine the client's wishes for end-of-life nursing care? Select all that apply.

❏ **1** Preferred place for death
❏ **2** Client expectations for nursing care
❏ **3** Financial responsibilities for the funeral
❏ **4** Where the funeral and burial will take place
❏ **5** Use of and the level of life-sustaining measures
❏ **6** Expectations regarding pain control and symptom management

Answer: 1, 2, 5, 6

Rationale: A nurse must assess the client's wishes for end-of-life nursing care, since these can influence how the nurse sets priorities for nursing diagnoses and plans and implements care. End-of-life assessment related to nursing care should include the preferred place for death; client expectations for nursing care; the use of and the level of life-sustaining measures; and expectations regarding pain control and symptom management. Financial responsibilities for the funeral and where the funeral and burial will take place are issues that the client may want to discuss, but they are unrelated to nursing care.

Test-Taking Strategy: Focus on the strategic words *end-of-life nursing care.* Read each option and select those that relate to nursing care. Financial responsibilities for the funeral and where the funeral and burial will take place are unrelated to nursing care. Review end-of-life nursing care issues if you had difficulty with this question.

Level of Cognitive Ability: Analysis
Client Needs: Psychosocial Integrity
Integrated Process: Nursing Process/Assessment
Content Area: Psychosocial Adaptation

Reference
Potter P, Perry A: *Fundamentals of nursing,* ed 6, St Louis, 2005, Mosby, p 578.

Multiple Response

77. A community health nurse is conducting an awareness workshop on adolescent suicide. Which of the following should the nurse discuss as risk factors? Select all that apply.

❑ **1** Family violence
❑ **2** Poor impulse control
❑ **3** Use of alcohol or drugs
❑ **4** Strong peer relationships
❑ **5** Family history of depression
❑ **6** Adequate school performance

Answer: 1, 2, 3, 5

Rationale: Risk factors for suicide among adolescents are depression; a family history of mental health disorders, especially depression and suicide; previous attempts at suicide; family violence or abuse; substance abuse; poor impulse control; poor school performance; feelings of worthlessness or hopelessness; and homosexuality.

Test-Taking Strategy: Focus on the subject, the risk factors for suicide. Noting the words *strong* in option 4 and *adequate* in option 6 will assist in eliminating these options as risk factors. Review risk factors for suicide in an adolescent if you had difficulty with this question.

Level of Cognitive Ability: Analysis
Client Needs: Psychosocial Integrity
Integrated Process: Nursing Process/Assessment
Content Area: Mental Health Disorders

Reference
McKinney E, James S, Murray S, et al: *Maternal-child nursing,* ed 2, Philadelphia, 2005, Saunders, p 1537.

Multiple Response

78. The nurse prepares to implement suicide precautions for an acutely suicidal client. Select the nursing interventions with regard to these precautions. Select all that apply.

❑ **1** Maintain arm's length distance with the client at all times.

❑ **2** Ensure that meal trays contain no glass or metal silverware.

❑ **3** Carefully watch the client swallow each dose of medication.

❑ **4** Conduct one-on-one nursing observation and interaction 24 hours a day.

❑ **5** Document client's mood, verbatim statements, and behaviors every 15 to 30 minutes per protocol.

❑ **6** Allow the client to totally cover self with the bedcovers during sleep at night as long as the nurse is present.

Answer: 1, 2, 3, 4, 5

Rationale: Suicide precautions involve constant observation of the client by the nursing staff. This intense attention from the nurse provides for safety and also allows for constant reassessment of risk. Suicide precautions include conducting one-on-one nursing observation and interaction 24 hours a day; maintaining arm's length distance with the client at all times; documenting client's mood, verbatim statements, and behaviors every 15 to 30 minutes per protocol; ensuring that meal trays contain no glass or metal silverware; carefully watching the client swallow each dose of medication; and explaining to the client the procedures involved with suicide precautions. During observation when the client is sleeping, the client's hands should always be in view and not under the bedcovers.

Test-Taking Strategy: Focus on the subject, suicide precautions, and note the strategic words *an acutely suicidal client.* Read each option carefully, keeping safety in mind. The only option that presents a risk is option 6, allowing the client to totally cover self with the bedcovers during sleep at night. Remember the client's hands should always be in view. Review nursing interventions related to suicide precautions if you had difficulty with this question.

Level of Cognitive Ability: Application
Client Needs: Psychosocial Integrity
Integrated Process: Nursing Process/Implementation
Content Area: Mental Health Disorders

Reference
Varcarolis E, Carson V, Shoemaker N: *Foundations of psychiatric mental health nursing,* ed 5, Philadelphia, 2006, Saunders, p 481.

Multiple Response

79. A client with a serious ulcer of the right foot is told that a right leg amputation may be necessary. The nurse monitors the client for which signs that are indicative of anticipatory grief? Select all that apply.

- ❑ **1** Periods of weeping or raging
- ❑ **2** Stating a fear of the future and unknown
- ❑ **3** Expressing anger at the medical professionals
- ❑ **4** Expressing a feeling of unreality and disbelief
- ❑ **5** Expressing a desire to run away from the situation
- ❑ **6** Stating that he does not need to know any details about his care

Answer: 1, 2, 3, 4, 5

Rationale: Anticipatory grief refers to the intellectual and emotional responses and behaviors by which individuals, families, or communities work through the process of modifying self-concept based on the perception of potential loss. Signs of anticipatory grief include feelings of emptiness or of being lost, a sense of being numb and fatigued, a feeling of unreality and disbelief, periods of weeping or raging, a desire to run away from the situation, a need to oversee every detail of care, fears of the future and the unknown, anger at medical professionals, pronounced clinging to or dependency on other family members, and fear of going crazy.

Test-Taking Strategy: Focus on the subject, the signs of anticipatory grief. Recall that anticipatory grief involves the intellectual and emotional responses and behaviors by which an individual works through the process of modifying self-concept based on the perception of potential loss. Read each option, keeping the subject of the question and the definition of anticipatory grief in mind to assist in answering correctly. Review these signs if you had difficulty with this question.

Level of Cognitive Ability: Analysis
Client Needs: Psychosocial Integrity
Integrated Process: Nursing Process/Assessment
Content Area: Psychosocial Adaptation

Reference
Varcarolis E, Carson V, Shoemaker N: *Foundations of psychiatric mental health nursing*, ed 5, Philadelphia, 2006, Saunders, p 608.

Multiple Response

80. A nurse manager is conducting an educational session for nursing staff on seclusion for clients with a mental health disorder. Under which circumstances is seclusion contraindicated? Select all that apply.

❏ 1 The client requests to be secluded.
❏ 2 The client has severe suicidal tendencies.
❏ 3 The client experienced a severe drug overdose.
❏ 4 The client presents a clear and present danger to self or others.
❏ 5 The client has been legally detained for involuntary treatment and is thought to pose an escape risk.
❏ 6 The client has an unstable mental health disorder and nursing staff needs to attend a monthly staff meeting.

Answer: 2, 3, 6

Rationale: Seclusion is the confinement of a client to a room in which the client is prevented from leaving. General contraindications to seclusion include extremely unstable medical or mental health conditions, delirium or dementia leading to inability to tolerate decreased stimulation, severe suicidal tendencies, severe drug reactions or overdoses or the need for close monitoring of drug doses, and desire for punishment of the client or convenience of the staff. Seclusion may be used for the following circumstances: the client presents a clear and present danger to self or others; the client has been legally detained for involuntary treatment and is thought to pose an escape risk; and the client requests to be secluded.

Test-Taking Strategy: Focus on the subject, contraindications to seclusion. Noting the word *severe* in options 2 and 3 will assist in selecting these options. Noting that option 6 indicates that seclusion is needed for the convenience of the nursing staff will assist in selecting this option. Review the reasons for and the contraindications to seclusion if you had difficulty with this question.

Level of Cognitive Ability: Analysis
Client Needs: Psychosocial Integrity
Integrated Process: Nursing Process/Analysis
Content Area: Mental Health Disorders

Reference
Varcarolis E, Carson V, Shoemaker N: *Foundations of psychiatric mental health nursing*, ed 5, Philadelphia, 2006, Saunders, pp 124, 496-497.

Multiple Response

81. A nurse implements deescalation techniques with a client who is extremely angry and exhibiting increasingly agitated behavior. Which deescalation techniques should the nurse employ? Select all that apply.

❑ **1** Avoid verbal struggles.
❑ **2** Place an arm around the client's shoulder.
❑ **3** Provide several clear options to the client.
❑ **4** Maintain the client's self-esteem and dignity.
❑ **5** Establish what the client considers to be his or her need.
❑ **6** Use a firm and aggressive tone of voice when speaking to the client.

Answer: 1, 3, 4, 5

Rationale: When the client is angry and exhibits increasingly agitated behavior, the nurse should employ deescalation techniques to prevent client violence and assaultive behaviors. These techniques include assessing the situation, using a calm and clear tone of voice when communicating with the client, remaining calm, and maintaining the client's self-esteem and dignity. The nurse should establish what the client considers to be his or her need and maintain a large personal space (touching the client could increase agitation). The nurse should also present several clear options to the client and avoid verbal struggles.

Test-Taking Strategy: Focus on the data and the subject of the question, deescalation techniques. Visualize each option to determine if the technique would calm or further agitate the client. Remember the need to maintain a calm approach and a large distance from the client. Review these deescalation techniques if you had difficulty with this question.

Level of Cognitive Ability: Application
Client Needs: Psychosocial Integrity
Integrated Process: Nursing Process/Implementation
Content Area: Mental Health Disorders

Reference
Varcarolis E, Carson V, Shoemaker N: *Foundations of psychiatric mental health nursing,* ed 5, Philadelphia, 2006, Saunders, p 496.

Multiple Response

82. A nurse is preparing a plan of care for a client diagnosed with acute mania. Identify appropriate nursing interventions that should be included in the plan of care. Select all that apply.

- ❏ **1** Place the client in seclusion.
- ❏ **2** Ignore any client complaints.
- ❏ **3** Use a firm and calm approach.
- ❏ **4** Use short and concise explanations and statements.
- ❏ **5** Remain neutral and avoid power struggles and value judgments.
- ❏ **6** Firmly redirect energy into more appropriate and constructive channels.

Answer: 3, 4, 5, 6

Rationale: A client with acute mania will be extremely restless, disorganized, and chaotic. Grandiose plans are extremely out of synch with reality, and judgment is poor. Interventions for the client in acute mania include using a firm and calm approach to provide structure and control, using short and concise explanations or statements because of the client's short attention span, remaining neutral and avoiding power struggles and value judgments, being consistent in approach and expectations and having frequent staff meetings to plan consistent approaches and to set agreed-on limits to avoid manipulation by the client, hearing and acting on legitimate client complaints, and redirecting energy into more appropriate and constructive channels.

Test-Taking Strategy: Focus on the subject, a client with acute mania. Read each option and think about the manifestations that occur in the client with acute mania and how the intervention may or may not assist the client. Eliminate option 1 because of the word *seclusion* and option 2 because of the word *ignore*. Review the interventions for the client with acute mania if you had difficulty with this question.

Level of Cognitive Ability: Application
Client Needs: Psychosocial Integrity
Integrated Process: Nursing Process/Implementation
Content Area: Mental Health Disorders

Reference
Varcarolis E, Carson V, Shoemaker N: *Foundations of psychiatric mental health nursing,* ed 5, Philadelphia, 2006, Saunders, p 369.

Multiple Response

83. A nurse is administering medication to a client who has just been told that he has inoperable pancreatic cancer when the client begins to cry. The nurse should take which appropriate therapeutic actions at this time? Select all that apply.

❑ **1** Call the client's spouse.
❑ **2** State to the client, "Tell me what you are feeling."
❑ **3** State to the client, "What are you thinking right now?"
❑ **4** Leave the client and close the door to the client's room.
❑ **5** Sit at the client's bedside and provide tissues to the client.
❑ **6** Ask the client if he would like the physician called for an order for a tranquilizer.

Answer: 2, 3, 5

Rationale: If a client begins to cry, the nurse should stay with the client, provide tissues as appropriate, and reinforce that it is all right to cry. Often, crying occurs at the time that feelings are closest to the surface and can be best identified. The nurse should encourage the client to express his thoughts and feelings. Calling the client's spouse is not an appropriate action unless the client makes this request. It is inappropriate to ask the client if he would like the physician called for an order for a tranquilizer; other interventions should be taken before medication is given. Additionally, this option does not address the client's feelings.

Test-Taking Strategy: Focus on the subject, the use of therapeutic communication techniques, which center on the client's feelings and concerns. This will direct you to the correct options. Review these therapeutic communication techniques if you had difficulty with this question.

Level of Cognitive Ability: Application
Client Needs: Psychosocial Integrity
Integrated Process: Caring
Content Area: Psychosocial Adaptation

Reference
Varcarolis E, Carson V, Shoemaker N: *Foundations of psychiatric mental health nursing,* ed 5, Philadelphia, 2006, Saunders, p 176.

Multiple Response

84. A client states to the nurse, "I want to kill myself." The nurse should take which appropriate actions? Select all that apply.

❑ **1** Ask the client if he has a plan to kill himself.

❑ **2** State to the client, "You don't really mean that."

❑ **3** State to the client, "We all have bad days and feel like killing ourselves."

❑ **4** Discuss with the client the feelings and circumstances that led to this decision.

❑ **5** Tell the client that this is a serious statement and that the information needs to be shared with other staff.

❑ **6** State to the client, "Killing yourself is not the answer to your problems, whatever they may be. Think how your children will feel."

Answer: 1, 4, 5

Rationale: If a client states to the nurse that he wants to kill himself, the nurse immediately assesses whether the client has a plan and the lethality of the plan. The nurse tells the client that this is serious, that the nurse does not want harm to come to the client, and that this information needs to be shared with other staff. The nurse also discusses with the client the feelings and circumstances that led to this decision. Option 2 devalues the client's feelings. Options 3 and 6 are also nontherapeutic and do not focus on the client's feelings.

Test-Taking Strategy: Focus on the subject, therapeutic communication techniques, which center on the client's feelings and concerns, and also keep in mind the seriousness of the client's statement. This will direct you to the correct options. Review therapeutic communication techniques and immediate interventions for a client who expresses suicidal intent if you had difficulty with this question.

Level of Cognitive Ability: Application
Client Needs: Psychosocial Integrity
Integrated Process: Communication and Documentation
Content Area: Psychosocial Adaptation

Reference
Varcarolis E, Carson V, Shoemaker N: *Foundations of psychiatric mental health nursing,* ed 5, Philadelphia, 2006, Saunders, p 176.

Multiple Response

85. The nurse expects to note which manifestations on assessment of a client with a diagnosis of bulimia nervosa? Select all that apply.

- ❏ **1** Dental caries
- ❏ **2** Reports of laxative abuse
- ❏ **3** Parotid gland enlargement
- ❏ **4** Reports of regular menses
- ❏ **5** Body weight 15% below expected weight
- ❏ **6** Hypokalemia as noted on the laboratory result form

Answer: 1, 2, 3, 6

Rationale: Bulimia nervosa is a condition characterized by a craving for food, often resulting in episodes of continuous eating followed by purging (self-induced vomiting), use of laxatives and/or diuretics, depression, and self-starvation. The client has a persistent overconcern with body weight and shape. Weight is maintained at or slightly below expected weight. Enlargement of the parotid glands occurs with dental erosion and caries as a result of the induced vomiting. Electrolyte imbalances are present as a result of abuse of laxatives or diuretics. Amenorrhea or irregular menses is reported.

Test-Taking Strategy: Focus on the client's diagnosis. Read each option carefully and think about the description of bulimia nervosa to select the correct options. Review the manifestations of bulimia nervosa if you had difficulty with this question.

Level of Cognitive Ability: Analysis
Client Needs: Psychosocial Integrity
Integrated Process: Nursing Process/Assessment
Content Area: Mental Health Disorders

References

Mosby's medical, nursing, and allied health dictionary, ed 7, St Louis, 2006, Mosby, p 268.
Stuart G, Laraia M: *Principles and practice of psychiatric nursing*, ed 7, St Louis, 2005, Mosby, p 528.
Varcarolis E, Carson V, Shoemaker N: *Foundations of psychiatric mental health nursing*, ed 5, Philadelphia, 2006, Saunders, p 304.

REFERENCES

Fortinash K, Holoday-Worret P: *Psychiatric mental health nursing,* ed 3, St Louis, 2004, Mosby.

McKinney E, James S, Murray S, et al: *Maternal-child nursing,* ed 2, Philadelphia, 2005, Saunders.

Mosby's medical, nursing, and allied health dictionary, ed 6, St Louis, 2006, Mosby.

Murray S, McKinney E: *Foundations of maternal-newborn nursing,* ed 4, Philadelphia, 2006, Saunders.

National Council of State Boards of Nursing: www.ncsbn.org.

National Council of State Boards of Nursing: *National Council of State Boards of Nursing test plan for the NCLEX-RN® Examination* (effective date: April 2007), Chicago, 2006, The Council.

Potter P, Perry A: *Fundamentals of nursing,* ed 6, St Louis, 2005, Mosby.

Stuart G, Laraia M: *Principles and practice of psychiatric nursing,* ed 7, St Louis, 2005, Mosby.

Varcarolis E, Carson V, Shoemaker N: *Foundations of psychiatric mental health nursing,* ed 5, Philadelphia, 2006, Saunders.

CHAPTER **5** ▲▲▲

Physiological Integrity Questions

The Physiological Integrity category of Client Needs includes four subcategories: Basic Care and Comfort, Pharmacological and Parenteral Therapies, Reduction of Risk Potential, and Physiological Adaptation. According to the National Council of State Boards of Nursing (NCSBN), Basic Care and Comfort accounts for 6% to 12% of the questions on the examination, Pharmacological and Parenteral Therapies make up 13% to 19% of the questions, Reduction of Risk Potential accounts for 13% to 19% of the questions, and Physiological Adaptation accounts for 11% to 17% of the questions (Box 5-1). Following is a description of each subcategory and its associated content. Also refer to the *National Council of State Boards of Nursing Test Plan for the NCLEX-RN® Examination* (2006) on the NCSBN website at www.ncsbn.org for additional information. Practice questions that address content in each subcategory follow the descriptions.

Basic Care and Comfort

Basic Care and Comfort questions (6% to 12%) test the knowledge, skill, and ability required to provide comfort and assistance to the client in the performance of activities of daily living. Some of the content related to this subcategory is identified in Box 5-2.

BOX 5-1 ▲ PHYSIOLOGICAL INTEGRITY

Basic Care and Comfort = 6% to 12% of the questions

Pharmacological and Parenteral Therapies = 13% to 19% of the questions

Reduction of Risk Potential = 13% to 19% of the questions

Physiological Adaptation = 11% to 17% of the questions

BOX 5-2 ▲ BASIC CARE AND COMFORT CONTENT

- Maintaining hygiene
- Maintaining nutrition and oral hydration
- Managing mobility and effects of immobility
- Monitoring elimination patterns
- Providing nonpharmacological interventions to provide comfort
- Providing rest and sleep
- Using alternative and complementary therapies
- Using assistive devices

Pharmacological and Parenteral Therapies

Pharmacological and Parenteral Therapies questions (13% to 19%) test the knowledge, skill, and ability required to administer medications and parenteral therapies. Some of the content related to this subcategory is identified in Box 5-3.

Reduction of Risk Potential

Reduction of Risk Potential questions (13% to 19%) test the knowledge, skill, and ability required to prevent complications or health problems related to the client's condition or any prescribed treatments or procedures. Some of the content related to this subcategory is identified in Box 5-4.

BOX 5-3 ▲ PHARMACOLOGICAL AND PARENTERAL THERAPIES CONTENT

- Administering blood products
- Administering intravenous therapy and parenteral fluids
- Administering medications
- Administering parenteral nutrition
- Caring for central venous access devices
- Identifying the contraindications and interactions associated with medications
- Monitoring for the intended effects of medications
- Monitoring for side effects, and adverse effects of medications
- Performing dosage calculations
- Providing pharmacological pain management

BOX 5-4 ▲ REDUCTION OF RISK POTENTIAL CONTENT

- Assisting with diagnostic tests and laboratory values
- Measuring vital signs
- Monitoring conscious sedation
- Monitoring for alterations in body systems
- Monitoring for complications of diagnostic tests and surgical and nonsurgical treatments and procedures
- Performing focused assessments
- Providing therapeutic procedures

Physiological Adaptation

Physiological Adaptation questions (11% to 17%) test the knowledge, skill, and ability required to provide care to clients with acute, chronic, or life-threatening conditions. Some of the content related to this subcategory is identified in Box 5-5.

BOX 5-5 ▲ PHYSIOLOGICAL ADAPTATION CONTENT

- Caring for the individual with an infectious disease
- Identifying unexpected responses to therapy
- Managing illness
- Monitoring for alterations in body systems
- Monitoring for fluid and electrolyte imbalances
- Taking action in medical emergencies
- Teaching the client about radiation therapy
- Understanding the pathophysiology of disease

Portions copyright by National Council of State Boards of Nursing, Inc. All rights reserved.

PRACTICE QUESTIONS

Multiple Response

86. A nurse provides information to a client who will be receiving relaxation therapy. The nurse tells the client that which effects occur from this type of therapy? Select all that apply.

- ❏ **1** Increased heart rate
- ❏ **2** Improved well-being
- ❏ **3** Lowered blood pressure
- ❏ **4** Increased respiratory rate
- ❏ **5** Decreased muscle tension
- ❏ **6** Increased neural impulses to the brain

Answer: 2, 3, 5

Rationale: Relaxation is the state of generalized decreased cognitive, physiological, and/or behavioral arousal. Relaxation elongates the muscle fibers, reduces the neural impulses to the brain, and thus decreases the activity of the brain and other systems. The effects of relaxation therapy include lowered heart rate, respiratory rate, and blood pressure; decreased muscle tension; improved well-being; and reduced symptom distress in persons experiencing complications from medical treatment or disease or grieving the loss of a significant other.

Test-Taking Strategy: Focus on the subject, the effects of relaxation therapy. Thinking about the definition of relaxation and recalling that it is the state of generalized decreased cognitive, physiological, and/or behavioral arousal will assist in directing you to the correct options. Review the effects of relaxation therapy if you had difficulty with this question.

Level of Cognitive Ability: Application
Client Needs: Physiological Integrity
Integrated Process: Teaching and Learning
Content Area: Basic Care and Comfort

Reference
Potter P, Perry A: *Fundamentals of nursing,* ed 6, St Louis, 2005, Mosby, p 916.

Chart/Exhibit with a Fill-in-the-Blank

87. The nurse reviews the client's vital signs in the client's chart. Based on these data, document the client's pulse pressure.

Answer: _____

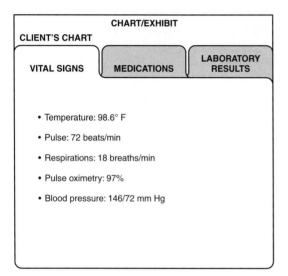

CHART/EXHIBIT

CLIENT'S CHART

| VITAL SIGNS | MEDICATIONS | LABORATORY RESULTS |

- Temperature: 98.6° F
- Pulse: 72 beats/min
- Respirations: 18 breaths/min
- Pulse oximetry: 97%
- Blood pressure: 146/72 mm Hg

Answer: 74

Rationale: The difference between the systolic and diastolic blood pressure is the pulse pressure. Therefore, if the client has a blood pressure of 146/72 mm Hg, then the pulse pressure is 74.

Test-Taking Strategy: Recall that the pulse pressure is the difference between the systolic and diastolic blood pressure, and then use simple mathematics to subtract 72 from 146 to yield 74. Review the procedure for determining the pulse pressure if you had difficulty with this question.

Level of Cognitive Ability: Application
Client Needs: Physiological Integrity
Integrated Process: Communication and Documentation
Content Area: Reduction of Risk Potential

Reference
Potter P, Perry A: *Fundamentals of nursing,* ed 6, St Louis, 2005, Mosby, p 653.

Multiple Response

88. The nurse should consider which of the following when determining whether a client could tolerate and benefit from active progressive relaxation? Select all that apply.

- ❑ **1** Social status
- ❑ **2** Financial status
- ❑ **3** Functional status
- ❑ **4** Medical diagnosis
- ❑ **5** Ability to expend energy
- ❑ **6** Motivation of the individual

Answer: 3, 4, 5, 6

Rationale: Active progressive relaxation training teaches the client how to effectively rest and reduce tension in the body. Some important considerations when choosing the type of relaxation technique is the client's physiological and psychological status. The client needs to be motivated to participate in this form of alternative therapy to obtain beneficial results. Because active progressive relaxation training requires a moderate expenditure of energy, the nurse needs to consider the client's medical diagnosis, functional status, and ability to expend energy. For example, a client with advanced respiratory disease may not have sufficient energy reserves to participate in active progressive relaxation techniques. The client's social or financial status has no relationship to his or her ability to tolerate and benefit from active progressive relaxation.

Test-Taking Strategy: Focus on the subject, determining whether a client could tolerate and benefit from active progressive relaxation. Use teaching-learning principles to determine that client motivation is a key factor in the learning process (option 6). From the remaining options, noting the strategic word *active* will assist in determining that options 3, 4, and 5 need to be considered. Review the characteristics of active progressive relaxation if you had difficulty with this question.

Level of Cognitive Ability: Analysis
Client Needs: Physiological Integrity
Integrated Process: Nursing Process/Assessment
Content Area: Basic Care and Comfort

Reference
Potter P, Perry A: *Fundamentals of nursing,* ed 6, St Louis, 2005, Mosby, pp 916-917.

Multiple Response

89. Which complementary and alternative therapies would be beneficial to induce relaxation for a client with advanced lung cancer? Select all that apply.

- ❏ **1** Biofeedback
- ❏ **2** Acupuncture
- ❏ **3** Herbal therapy
- ❏ **4** Passive relaxation
- ❏ **5** Creative visualization
- ❏ **6** Active progressive relaxation

Answer: 4, 5

Rationale: Some important considerations when choosing the type of relaxation techniques are the client's physiological and psychological status. Clients with advanced disease such as lung cancer may seek relaxation training to reduce their stress response. However, techniques such as active progressive relaxation training require a moderate expenditure of energy, which can amplify a person's fatigue and limit his or her ability to complete individual relaxation sessions and practice. Therefore active progressive relaxation would not be appropriate for a client with advanced lung disease who has decreased energy reserves. Passive relaxation involves teaching a client to relax individual muscle groups passively and is a useful technique for the client for whom the effort and energy expenditure of active muscle contraction lead to discomfort or exhaustion. Creative visualization is a form of self-directed imagery based on the principle of mind-body connectivity and does not require energy expenditure. Biofeedback is a group of therapeutic procedures that use electronic or electromechanical instruments to measure, process, and provide information to the client about his or her neuromuscular and autonomic nervous system activity. This procedure is a training-specific therapy and requires energy expenditure and client participation and would not be the best measure for a client with advanced lung disease. Acupuncture is a method of stimulating certain points (acupoints) on the body by inserting special needles to modify the perception of pain, normalize physiological function, or treat or prevent disease. It is an invasive procedure and does not focus specifically on relaxation. Herbal therapy is also an invasive therapy and does not specifically focus on relaxation. Additionally, physician's approval should be obtained before using herbal therapy.

Test-Taking Strategy: Focus on the subject, measures to produce relaxation, and the client's diagnosis. Eliminate options 2 and 3 because they are invasive and do not specifically focus on relaxation. Next eliminate options 1 and 6 because they require effort and energy expenditure, and a client with decreased energy reserves would be unable to participate in these measures. Review these types of complementary and alternative therapies if you had difficulty with this question.

Level of Cognitive Ability: Application
Client Needs: Physiological Integrity
Integrated Process: Nursing Process/Implementation
Content Area: Basic Care and Comfort

Reference
Potter P, Perry A: *Fundamentals of nursing*, ed 6, St Louis, 2005, Mosby, pp 917-923.

Prioritizing (Ordered Response)

90. A client with weakness of the right leg has an order for a single straight-legged cane for ambulation, and the nurse instructs the client in the use of the cane. Arrange the following actions in the appropriate order for preparing and instructing the client about the use of the cane. (Number 1 is the first action and number 6 is the last action.)

___ Measure the cane for the correct height.

___ Inform the client about the physician's order.

___ Instruct the client to move the weaker leg forward.

___ Instruct the client to move the stronger leg forward.

___ Instruct the client to hold the cane on the strong side of the body.

___ Instruct the client to place the cane forward 15 to 25 cm (6 to 10 inches), keeping the body weight on both legs.

Answer: 2, 1, 5, 6, 3, 4

Rationale: The single straight-legged cane is used to support and balance a client with decreased leg strength. The nurse would first inform the client about the physician's order for walking with a cane and then would measure the cane to ensure that it is an appropriate and safe height. The cane should be held on the stronger side of the body. For maximum support when walking, the client places the cane forward 15 to 25 cm (6 to 10 inches), keeping body weight on both legs. The weaker leg is moved forward to the cane so that body weight is divided between the cane and the stronger leg. The stronger leg is then advanced past the cane so that the weaker leg and the body weight are supported by the cane and stronger leg. While walking, the client continually repeats these steps. The client must be taught that two points of support, such as both feet or one foot and the cane, are present at all times.

Test-Taking Strategy: Remember that it is always important to inform the client of the treatment plan before implementing the plan. Next the nurse needs to ensure safety by measuring the height of the cane for the client. To select the order of action from the remaining options, visualize the procedure for ambulating with a cane. Review this procedure if you had difficulty with this question.

Level of Cognitive Ability: Application
Client Needs: Physiological Integrity
Integrated Process: Teaching and Learning
Content Area: Basic Care and Comfort

Reference
Potter P, Perry A: *Fundamentals of nursing,* ed 6, St Louis, 2005, Mosby, p 948.

Figure/Illustration with a Multiple Choice

91. The nurse looks at a hospitalized client's cardiac monitor screen and notes this cardiac rhythm (refer to figure). The nurse prepares to administer which priority measure?

❑ 1 Defibrillation
❑ 2 Measurement of vital signs
❑ 3 Insertion of an endotracheal tube
❑ 4 Administration of antidysrhythmic medication

Answer: 1

Rationale: The goal of treatment for ventricular fibrillation (VF) is to terminate the VF immediately. Therefore, if the client experiences VF, the priority is to defibrillate the client immediately. If the VF does not terminate after three rapid successive shocks of increasing energy, the nurse and resuscitation team must resume cardiopulmonary resuscitation and provide airway management via oxygen and antidysrhythmic therapy. If VF is successfully converted to an organized rhythm, the nurse continues supportive therapy and assists the physician in treating potential causes of VF and preventing its recurrence. Measurement of vital signs is not the priority intervention, although it is part of monitoring during supportive therapy. An endotracheal tube may or may not be needed.

Test-Taking Strategy: Focus on the cardiac rhythm and note that it indicates VF. Remember, when the client experiences *fibrillation*, the client must be *defibrillated*. Review the characteristics of this rhythm and its priority treatment if you had difficulty with this question.

Level of Cognitive Ability: Application
Client Needs: Physiological Integrity
Integrated Process: Nursing Process/Implementation
Content Area: Physiological Adaptation

Reference
Ignatavicius D, Workman M: *Medical surgical nursing: critical thinking for collaborative care,* ed 5, Philadelphia, 2006, Saunders, pp 731-732.

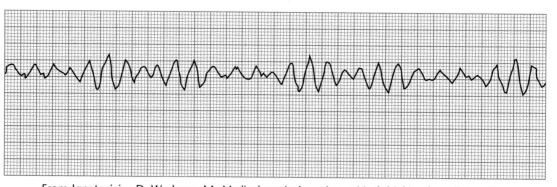

From Ignatavicius D, Workman M: *Medical surgical nursing: critical thinking for collaborative care,* ed 5, Philadelphia, 2006, Saunders.

Multiple Response

92. A nurse is caring for a client who is receiving blood transfusion therapy. Which clinical manifestations would alert the nurse to a hemolytic transfusion reaction? Select all that apply.

- ❏ **1** Headache
- ❏ **2** Tachycardia
- ❏ **3** Hypertension
- ❏ **4** Apprehension
- ❏ **5** Distended neck veins
- ❏ **6** A sense of impending doom

Answer: 1, 2, 3, 4, 6

Rationale: Hemolytic transfusion reactions are caused by blood type or Rh incompatibility. When blood containing antigens different from the client's own antigens is infused, antigen-antibody complexes are formed in the client's blood. These complexes destroy the transfused cells and start inflammatory responses in the client's blood vessel walls and organs. The reaction may be mild, with fever and chills, or life threatening, with disseminated intravascular coagulation and circulatory collapse. Other manifestations include apprehension, headache, chest pain, low back pain, tachycardia, tachypnea, hypotension, hemoglobinuria, and a sense of impending doom. The onset may be immediate or may not occur until subsequent units have been transfused. A bounding pulse and distended neck veins are characteristics of circulatory overload.

Test-Taking Strategy: Focus on the subject, a hemolytic transfusion reaction. Recall the pathophysiology of this type of reaction to select the correct options. Also think about other types of transfusion reactions that can occur, and recall that a bounding pulse and distended neck veins are characteristic of circulatory overload. Review the clinical manifestations of a hemolytic transfusion reaction if you had difficulty with this question.

Level of Cognitive Ability: Analysis
Client Needs: Physiological Integrity
Integrated Process: Nursing Process/Assessment
Content Area: Pharmacological and Parenteral Therapies

Reference
Ignatavicius D, Workman M: *Medical surgical nursing: critical thinking for collaborative care,* ed 5, Philadelphia, 2006, Saunders, p 916.

Prioritizing (Ordered Response)

93. A nurse is teaching a client unable to bear weight on one leg how to ascend stairs with crutches. From the following, arrange the selected options in the appropriate order of instruction. (Number 1 is the first step and number 6 is the last step.)

—— Explain the procedure to the client.

—— Instruct the client to lift and place both crutches on the stairs.

—— Instruct the client to transfer the body weight to the crutches.

—— Instruct the client to shift the weight from the crutches to the unaffected leg.

—— Instruct the client to advance the unaffected leg between the crutches to the stairs.

—— Instruct the client to stand at the bottom of the stairs using a modified three-point gait.

Answer: 1, 6, 3, 5, 4, 2

Rationale: When ascending stairs on crutches, the client usually uses a modified three-point gait. The client stands at the bottom of the stairs and transfers body weight to the crutches. The unaffected leg is advanced between the crutches to the stairs. The client then shifts weight from the crutches to the unaffected leg. Finally, the client lifts both crutches and places them on the stairs. This sequence is repeated until the client reaches the top of the stairs. To descend the stairs, a three-phase sequence is also used. The client transfers body weight to the unaffected leg. The crutches are placed on the stairs, and the client begins to transfer body weight to the crutches, moving the affected leg forward. Finally, the unaffected leg is moved to the stairs with the crutches. Again, the client repeats the sequence until reaching the bottom of the stairs.

Test-Taking Strategy: Remember that the nurse always explains a procedure to a client before implementing the procedure. Next visualize the process of ascending stairs with crutches. Also remember the phrase *good up and bad down.* When going up the stairs, the client moves the good leg up first; when descending stairs, the client moves the bad leg down first. Review crutch-walking procedure on stairs if you had difficulty with this question.

Level of Cognitive Ability: Application
Client Needs: Physiological Integrity
Integrated Process: Teaching and Learning
Content Area: Basic Care and Comfort

Reference
Potter P, Perry A: *Fundamentals of nursing,* ed 6, St Louis, 2005, Mosby, p 951.

Figure/Illustration with a Multiple Choice

94. A child sustains a fractured humerus from a fall out of a tree house. The nurse provides a picture of the fracture for the child's parent and tells the parent that this type of fracture is known as which of the following? (Refer to figure.)

❑ **1** Spiral
❑ **2** Greenstick
❑ **3** Transverse
❑ **4** Comminuted

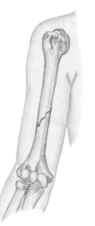

From McKinney E, James S, Murray S, et al: *Maternal-child nursing,* ed 2, Philadelphia, 2005, Saunders

Answer: 1

Rationale: A spiral fracture is characterized by a twisted or circular break that affects the length rather than the width. A greenstick fracture is a break that occurs through the periosteum on one side of the bone with only bowing or buckling on the other side. In a transverse fracture the break or fracture line occurs at right angles to the long axis of the bone. In a comminuted fracture the bone is splintered into pieces.

Test-Taking Strategy: Focus on the characteristics of the fracture in the figure. Note the relationship between the visual characteristics and the word *spiral*. Review the characteristics of the various types of fractures if you had difficulty with this question.

Level of Cognitive Ability: Analysis
Client Needs: Physiological Integrity
Integrated Process: Teaching and Learning
Content Area: Physiological Adaptation

Reference
McKinney E, James S, Murray S, et al: *Maternal-child nursing,* ed 2, Philadelphia, 2005, Saunders, p 1426.

Multiple Response

95. A nurse is assessing a pregnant client with a diagnosis of abruptio placenta. The nurse expects to note which manifestations of this condition? Select all that apply.

   ❑ 1 Uterine irritability
   ❑ 2 Uterine tenderness
   ❑ 3 Painless vaginal bleeding
   ❑ 4 Abdominal and low back pain
   ❑ 5 Strong and frequent contractions
   ❑ 6 Nonreassuring fetal heart rate patterns

Answer: 1, 2, 4, 6

Rationale: Abruptio placenta is the separation of a normally implanted placenta before the fetus is born. It occurs when there is bleeding and formation of a hematoma on the maternal side of the placenta. Manifestations include vaginal bleeding, aching and dull abdominal and low back pain, uterine irritability with frequent low-intensity contractions, uterine tenderness that may be localized to the site of the abruption, and a high uterine resting tone identified by the use of an intrauterine pressure catheter. Additional signs include nonreassuring fetal heart rate patterns, signs of hypovolemic shock, and fetal death.

Test-Taking Strategy: Focus on the diagnosis. Recalling the pathophysiology associated with this hemorrhagic condition will assist in selecting the correct options. Remember that abruptio placenta occurs when there is bleeding and formation of a hematoma on the maternal side of the placenta. Review the manifestations of abruptio placenta if you had difficulty with this question.

Level of Cognitive Ability: Analysis
Client Needs: Physiological Integrity
Integrated Process: Nursing Process/Assessment
Content Area: Physiological Adaptation

Reference
McKinney E, James S, Murray S, et al: *Maternal-child nursing,* ed 2, Philadelphia, 2005, Saunders, pp 625-626.

Multiple Response

96. Tranylcypromine (Parnate) is prescribed for a client with depression. The nurse instructs the client to avoid which food items? Select all that apply.

- ❏ **1** Figs
- ❏ **2** Apples
- ❏ **3** Bananas
- ❏ **4** Broccoli
- ❏ **5** Sauerkraut
- ❏ **6** Baked chicken

Answer: 1, 3, 5

Rationale: Tranylcypromine is a monoamine oxidase inhibitor (MAOI). Foods that contain tyramine need to be avoided because of the risk of hypertensive crisis associated with use of this medication. Foods to avoid include avocados; soybeans; sauerkraut; figs; meats or fish that are fermented, smoked, or otherwise aged; some cheeses; yeast extract; bananas; and some beers and wine.

Test-Taking Strategy: Focus on the name of the medication and recall that tranylcypromine is an MAOI. Next recall the foods that contain tyramine to answer the question. Remember that figs, bananas, and sauerkraut are high in tyramine. Review this medication and the foods high in tyramine if you had difficulty with this question.

Level of Cognitive Ability: Application
Client Needs: Physiological Integrity
Integrated Process: Teaching and Learning
Content Area: Pharmacological and Parenteral Therapies

Reference
Varcarolis E, Carson V, Shoemaker N: *Foundations of psychiatric mental health nursing,* ed 5, Philadelphia, 2006, Saunders, pp 349, 351.

Prioritizing (Ordered Response)

97. The nurse is counseling a client on using laxatives to manage constipation. Arrange all the following in the recommended stepwise progression for their use. (Number 1 is the first laxative that would be used, and number 6 is the last laxative that would be used.)

___ Enemas
___ Osmotics
___ Stimulants
___ Suppositories
___ Stool softeners
___ Bulk-forming laxatives

Answer: 6, 3, 4, 5, 2, 1

Rationale: Constipation is difficulty in passing stools or incomplete or infrequent passage of hard stools. Several interventions can be used to manage constipation, including increasing fluid intake; avoiding products such as coffee, tea, and alcohol because of their diuretic effect; eating high-fiber foods; and engaging in physical activity. If these conservative measures fail to manage the constipation, then it may be necessary to prescribe laxatives. Laxatives should be used with caution and in a stepwise progression: (1) bulk-forming laxatives, (2) stool softeners, (3) osmotics, (4) stimulants, (5) suppositories, and (6) enemas (used as a last resort). Bulk-forming laxatives are natural fibrous substances that promote large, soft stools by absorbing water into the intestine, increasing fecal bulk and peristalsis. Stool softeners are emollients that lower surface tension and promote water accumulation in the intestine and stool. Osmotics are hyperosmolar laxatives that pull water into the colon and increase water in the feces to increase bulk, which stimulates peristalsis. Stimulants increase peristalsis by irritating sensory nerve endings in the intestinal mucosa. An enema is the introduction of a solution into the rectum for cleansing.

Test-Taking Strategy: Focus on the subject, the recommended stepwise progression for the use of laxatives. Recall the action of each type of laxative identified in the options and arrange them in order from least invasive or irritating to the intestinal tract to most invasive. Review these various types of laxatives if you had difficulty with this question.

Level of Cognitive Ability: Application
Client Needs: Physiological Integrity
Integrated Process: Teaching and Learning
Content Area: Pharmacological and Parenteral Therapies

Reference
Potter P, Perry A: *Fundamentals of nursing*, ed 6, St Louis, 2005, Mosby, p 1394.

Multiple Response

98. A nurse is developing a care plan for a client with urge urinary incontinence. Which of the following interventions would be most helpful for this type of incontinence? Select all that apply.

❏ **1** Surgery
❏ **2** Bladder retraining
❏ **3** Scheduled toileting
❏ **4** Dietary modifications
❏ **5** Pelvic muscle exercises
❏ **6** Intermittent catheterization

Answer: 2, 3, 4, 5

Rationale: Urge incontinence is the involuntary passage of urine after a strong sense of the urgency to void. It is characterized by urinary urgency, often with frequency (more often than every 2 hours), bladder spasm or contraction, and voiding in either small amounts (less than 100 mL) or large amounts (greater than 500 mL). It can be caused by decreased bladder capacity, irritation of the bladder stretch receptors, infection, and alcohol or caffeine ingestion. Interventions to assist the client with urge incontinence include bladder retraining, scheduled toileting, dietary modifications such as eliminating alcohol and caffeine intake, and pelvic muscle exercises to strengthen the muscles. Surgery and urinary catheterization are invasive measures and will not assist in the treatment of urge incontinence.

Test-Taking Strategy: Focus on the subject, interventions that would be most helpful for urge urinary incontinence. Recalling the definition of this type of incontinence will assist in selecting the correct options. Also note that options 1 and 6 are invasive measures, and these types of measures are avoided. Review the interventions for urge urinary incontinence if you had difficulty with this question.

Level of Cognitive Ability: Application
Client Needs: Physiological Integrity
Integrated Process: Nursing Process/Planning
Content Area: Basic Care and Comfort

References
Harkreader H, Hogan MA: *Fundamentals of nursing: caring and clinical judgment,* ed 2, Philadelphia, 2004, Saunders, p 708.
Potter P, Perry A: *Fundamentals of nursing,* ed 6, St Louis, 2005, Mosby, p 1349.

Multiple Response

99. A nurse is performing a medication assessment of a client who has urinary elimination problems. From the following list of medications being taken by the client, identify those that interfere with elimination. Select all that apply.

- ❑ **1** Cefaclor (Ceclor)
- ❑ **2** Dicyclomine (Bentyl)
- ❑ **3** Imipramine (Tofranil)
- ❑ **4** Oxybutynin (Ditropan)
- ❑ **5** Levothyroxine (Synthroid)
- ❑ **6** Bethanechol chloride (Urecholine)

Answer: 2, 3, 4, 6

Rationale: Several types of medication can affect urinary elimination. Anticholinergics such as oxybutynin and antispasmodics such as dicyclomine decrease detrusor contractility and cause urinary retention and hesitancy. Tricyclic antidepressants such as imipramine also decrease detrusor contractility and cause urinary retention. Cholinergics such as bethanechol chloride increase detrusor contractility and cause urgency and incontinence. Other types of medications that affect urinary elimination include alpha-sympathomimetics, alpha-blockers, estrogens and antiandrogens, nonsteroidal anti-inflammatories, diuretics, aminoglycoside antibiotics, calcium channel blockers, and alcohol. Cefaclor is a second-generation cephalosporin. Levothyroxine is a thyroid medication.

Test-Taking Strategy: Focus on the subject, medications that affect urinary elimination. This is a difficult question; it is first necessary to know the classification of each medication in the options and then to recall those classifications that affect urinary elimination. Review these medications and classifications that affect urinary elimination if you had difficulty with this question.

Level of Cognitive Ability: Analysis
Client Needs: Physiological Integrity
Integrated Process: Nursing Process/Analysis
Content Area: Pharmacological and Parenteral Therapies

References
Black J, Hawks J: *Medical-surgical nursing: clinical management for positive outcomes,* ed 7, Philadelphia, 2005, Saunders, p 791.
Hodgson B, Kizior R: *Saunders nursing drug handbook 2007,* Philadelphia, 2007, Saunders, pp 195, 686.

Multiple Response

100. A nurse is performing range-of-motion (ROM) exercises on a client when the client unexpectedly develops spastic muscle contractions. The nurse should implement which interventions? Select all that apply.

- ❑ **1** Stop movement of affected part.
- ❑ **2** Massage affected part vigorously.
- ❑ **3** Notify the physician immediately.
- ❑ **4** Force movement of the joint supporting the muscle.
- ❑ **5** Ask the client to stand and walk rapidly around the room.
- ❑ **6** Place continuous gentle pressure on the muscle group until it relaxes.

Answer: 1, 6

Rationale: ROM exercises should put each joint through as full a range of motion as possible without causing discomfort. An unexpected outcome is the development of spastic muscle contraction during ROM exercises. If this occurs, the nurse should stop movement of the affected part and place continuous gentle pressure on the muscle group until it relaxes. Once the contraction subsides, the exercises are resumed using slower, steady movement. Massaging the affected part vigorously may worsen the contraction. There is no need to notify the physician unless intervention is ineffective. The nurse should never force movement of a joint. Asking the client to stand and walk rapidly around the room is an inappropriate measure. Additionally, if the client is able to walk, ROM exercises are probably unnecessary.

Test-Taking Strategy: Focus on the subject, interventions to relieve spastic muscle contractions. Eliminate option 2 because of the word *vigorously,* option 3 because of the word *immediately,* and option 4 because of the word *force.* Next eliminate option 5 because, if the client is able to walk, ROM exercises are probably unnecessary. Review the unexpected outcomes related to ROM exercises and their treatment if you had difficulty with this question.

Level of Cognitive Ability: Application
Client Needs: Physiological Integrity
Integrated Process: Nursing Process/Implementation
Content Area: Basic Care and Comfort

Reference
Potter P, Perry A: *Fundamentals of nursing,* ed 6, St Louis, 2005, Mosby, p 267.

Multiple Response

101. A nurse is getting a client out of bed for the first time after having abdominal surgery. What clinical manifestations would indicate to the nurse that the client may be experiencing orthostatic hypotension? Select all that apply.

- ❑ 1 Nausea
- ❑ 2 Dizziness
- ❑ 3 Bradycardia
- ❑ 4 Lightheadedness
- ❑ 5 Flushing of the face
- ❑ 6 Reports of seeing spots

Answer: 1, 2, 4, 6

Rationale: Orthostatic hypotension occurs when a normotensive person develops symptoms of low blood pressure when rising to an upright position. Whenever the nurse gets a client up and out of a bed or chair, there is a risk for orthostatic hypotension. Symptoms of dizziness, lightheadedness, nausea, tachycardia, pallor, and reports of seeing spots are characteristic of orthostatic hypotension. A drop of approximately 15 mm Hg in the systolic blood pressure and 10 mm Hg in the diastolic blood pressure also occurs. Fainting can result without intervention, which includes immediately assisting the client to a lying position.

Test-Taking Strategy: Focus on the subject, the manifestations of orthostatic hypotension. As you read each option, think about the physiological changes that occur when the blood pressure drops. This will assist in answering the question. Review the manifestations of orthostatic hypotension if you had difficulty with this question.

Level of Cognitive Ability: Analysis
Client Needs: Physiological Integrity
Integrated Process: Nursing Process/Assessment
Content Area: Physiological Adaptation

Reference
Potter P, Perry A: *Fundamentals of nursing,* ed 6, St Louis, 2005, Mosby, p 283.

Figure/Illustration with a Fill-in-the-Blank

102. The physician prescribes 250 mg of amikacin sulfate (Amikin) every 12 hours to treat a skin infection. The nurse prepares how many milliliters to administer one dose? (Refer to figure.)

Answer _____ **mL**

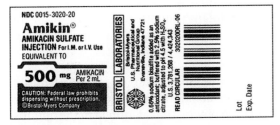

From Kee J, Marshall S: *Clinical calculations: with applications to general and specialty areas,* ed 5, Philadelphia, 2004, Saunders.

Answer: 1

Rationale: Use the medication calculation formula.

Formula

$$\frac{\text{Desired} \times \text{mL}}{\text{Available}} = \text{mL per dose}$$

$$\frac{250 \text{ mg} \times 2 \text{ mL}}{500 \text{ mg}} = 1 \text{ mL per dose}$$

Test-Taking Strategy: Focus on the data in the medication label. Follow the formula for calculating the correct dose. Once you have performed the calculation, recheck your work with a calculator and make sure that the answer makes sense. If you had difficulty with this question, review medication calculation problems.

Level of Cognitive Ability: Application
Client Needs: Physiological Integrity
Integrated Process: Nursing Process/Implementation
Content Area: Pharmacological and Parenteral Therapies

Reference
Kee J, Marshall S: *Clinical calculations: with applications to general and specialty areas,* ed 5, Philadelphia, 2004, Saunders, pp 80, 182.

Multiple Response

103. A nurse in the postpartum unit is assessing a newborn infant for signs of breastfeeding problems. Which of the following indicates a problem? Select all that apply.

❏ **1** The infant exhibits dimpling of the cheeks.

❏ **2** The infant makes smacking or clicking sounds.

❏ **3** The mother's breast gets softer during a feeding.

❏ **4** Milk drips from the mother's breast occasionally.

❏ **5** The infant falls asleep after feeding less than 5 minutes.

❏ **6** The infant can be heard swallowing frequently during a feeding.

Answer: 1, 2, 5

Rationale: It is important for the nurse to identify breast-feeding problems while the mother is hospitalized so that the nurse can teach the mother how to prevent and treat any problems. Infant signs of breastfeeding problems include falling asleep after feeding less than 5 minutes; refusing to breastfeed; tongue thrusting; making smacking or clicking sounds; dimpling of the cheeks; failing to open the mouth at latch-on; turning the lower lip in; making short, choppy motions of the jaw; and not swallowing audibly. Hearing the infant swallow, softening of the breast during feeding, and noting milk in the infant's mouth or dripping from the mother's breast occasionally are signs that the infant is receiving adequate nutrition.

Test-Taking Strategy: Focus on the subject, signs of breast-feeding problems. Think about the process of feeding and visualize the effect of each observation identified in the options. This will direct you to the correct options. Review the signs of breastfeeding problems if you had difficulty with this question.

Level of Cognitive Ability: Analysis
Client Needs: Physiological Integrity
Integrated Process: Nursing Process/Assessment
Content Area: Physiological Adaptation

Reference
McKinney E, James S, Murray S, et al: *Maternal-child nursing,* ed 2, Philadelphia, 2005, Saunders, p 583.

Multiple Response

104. A nurse is monitoring a client for behavioral indicators of the effects of pain. Which of the following are indicators that the client is in pain? Select all that apply.

- ❏ **1** Gasping
- ❏ **2** Lip biting
- ❏ **3** Muscle tension
- ❏ **4** Pacing activities
- ❏ **5** Conversing with the roommate
- ❏ **6** Enjoying social interaction with visitors

Answer 1, 2, 3, 4

Rationale: The nurse should assess verbalization, vocal response, facial and body movements, and social interaction as indicators of pain. Behavioral indicators of pain include moaning, crying, gasping, and grunting (vocalizations); grimacing, clenching teeth, wrinkling the forehead, tightly closing or widely opening the eyes or mouth, lip biting (facial expressions); restlessness, immobilization, muscle tension, increased hand and finger movements, pacing activities, rhythmic or rubbing motions, protective movements of body parts (body movement); avoidance of conversation, focusing only on activities for pain relief, avoiding social contacts and interactions, and reduced attention span.

Test-Taking Strategy: Focus on the subject, behavioral indicators of pain. Think about the physiological and psychosocial responses that occur during the pain experience as you read each option. This will assist in answering correctly. Review the behavioral indicators of pain if you had difficulty with this question.

Level of Cognitive Ability: Analysis
Client Needs: Physiological Integrity
Integrated Process: Nursing Process/Assessment
Content Area: Basic Care and Comfort

Reference
Potter P, Perry A: *Fundamentals of nursing*, ed 6, St Louis, 2005, Mosby, p 1245.

Prioritizing (Ordered Response)

105. A nurse is caring for a postoperative client who may begin taking oral nutrition. To ensure tolerance of the diet, arrange all the following in appropriate order of diet progression. (Number 1 is the first food that would be offered to the client [easiest to digest], and number 6 is the last food item that would be offered [most difficult to digest].)

___ Bananas
___ Vegetables
___ Orange juice
___ Scrambled eggs
___ Clear fruit juices
___ Moist, tender meats

Answer: 4, 6, 2, 3, 1, 5

Rationale: When a client begins to take oral nutrition, the diet should progress from food items that are easily digested to those that are more difficult to digest. The client should begin on a clear liquid diet (clear fruit juices) and progress to a full liquid diet (orange juice). If a full liquid diet is tolerated, then the client can progress to pureed-type foods (scrambled eggs) and then to soft foods (bananas). If these foods are tolerated, the client can progress to low-residue foods such as moist, tender meats and finally to higher fiber foods such as vegetables.

Test-Taking Strategy: Focus on the subject, diet progression when the client begins oral nutrition. Answer correctly by selecting the foods in order of how easily the body will digest them. This will direct you to the correct order of diet progression. Review diet progression if you had difficulty with this question.

Level of Cognitive Ability: Application
Client Needs: Physiological Integrity
Integrated Process: Nursing Process/Implementation
Content Area: Basic Care and Comfort

Reference
Potter P, Perry A: *Fundamentals of nursing,* ed 6, St Louis, 2005, Mosby, p 1298.

Multiple Response

106. A nurse is developing a care plan for a client receiving enteral nutrition and identifies the situations that place the client at risk for aspiration. Which of the following place the client at increased risk for aspiration? Select all that apply.

❏ **1** Sedation
❏ **2** Coughing
❏ **3** An artificial airway
❏ **4** Head elevated position
❏ **5** Nasotracheal suctioning
❏ **6** Decreased level of consciousness

Answer: 1, 2, 3, 5, 6

Rationale: A serious complication associated with enteral feedings is aspiration of formula into the tracheobronchial tree. Some common conditions that increase the risk for aspiration include coughing, nasotracheal suctioning, an artificial airway, sedation, decreased level of consciousness, and lying flat. A head elevated position does not increase the risk of aspiration.

Test-Taking Strategy: Focus on the subject, the risks associated with aspiration. Recall that aspiration is the inhalation of foreign material into the tracheobronchial tree. Next read each option and think about the effect it produces with regard to aspiration. This will direct you to the correct options. Review the risks associated with aspiration if you had difficulty with this question.

Level of Cognitive Ability: Analysis
Client Needs: Physiological Integrity
Integrated Process: Nursing Process/Analysis
Content Area: Basic Care and Comfort

Reference
Potter P, Perry A: *Fundamentals of nursing*, ed 6, St Louis, 2005, Mosby, p 1304.

Multiple Response

107. A nurse is counseling the family of a client who has terminal cancer about palliative care. The nurse explains that which of the following are goals of palliative care? Select all that apply.

❑ **1** Delays death
❑ **2** Offers a support system
❑ **3** Provides relief from pain
❑ **4** Enhances the quality of life
❑ **5** Focuses only on the client, not the family
❑ **6** Manages symptoms of disease and therapies

Answer: 2, 3, 4, 6

Rationale: Palliative care is a philosophy of total care. Palliative care goals include providing relief from pain and other distressing symptoms, affirming life and regarding dying as a normal process, neither hastening nor postponing death, integrating psychological and spiritual aspects of client care, offering a support system to help the client live as actively as possible until death, offering a support system to help families cope during the client's illness and their own bereavement, and enhancing the quality of life.

Test-Taking Strategy: Focus on the subject, goals of palliative care. Recall that palliative care interventions are designed to relieve or reduce the intensity of uncomfortable symptoms but not to produce a cure, and that palliative care is a philosophy of total care. With this in mind, read each option and determine if it meets this description. Review the goals of palliative care if you had difficulty with this question.

Level of Cognitive Ability: Application
Client Needs: Physiological Integrity
Integrated Process: Caring
Content Area: Basic Care and Comfort

Reference
Potter P, Perry A: *Fundamentals of nursing,* ed 6, St Louis, 2005, Mosby, pp 585-587.

Multiple Response

108. A nurse is caring for a client with a terminal condition who is dying. Which respiratory assessment findings would indicate to the nurse that death is imminent? Select all that apply.

- ❏ **1** Dyspnea
- ❏ **2** Cyanosis
- ❏ **3** Kussmaul's respiration
- ❏ **4** Tachypnea without apnea
- ❏ **5** Irregular respiratory pattern
- ❏ **6** Adventitious bubbling lung sounds

Answer: 1, 2, 5, 6

Rationale: Respiratory assessment findings that indicate death is imminent include altered patterns of respiration, such as slow, labored, irregular, or Cheyne-Stokes pattern (alternating periods of apnea and deep, rapid breathing); increased respiratory secretions and adventitious bubbling lung sounds (death rattle); irritation of the tracheobronchial airway as evidenced by hiccups, chest pain, fatigue, or exhaustion; and poor gas exchange as evidenced by hypoxia, dyspnea, or cyanosis. Kussmaul's respirations are abnormally deep, very rapid sighing respirations characteristic of diabetic ketoacidosis.

Test-Taking Strategy: Focus on the subject, respiratory assessment findings that indicate death is imminent. Think about the physiological processes that occur in the dying person as you read each option. This will assist in answering the question. Review these respiratory assessment findings if you had difficulty with this question.

Level of Cognitive Ability: Analysis
Client Needs: Physiological Integrity
Integrated Process: Nursing Process/Assessment
Content Area: Basic Care and Comfort

Reference
Harkreader H, Hogan MA: *Fundamentals of nursing: caring and clinical judgment,* ed 2, Philadelphia, 2004, Saunders, p 1119.

Multiple Response

109. A nurse is teaching a client about general hygienic measures for foot and nail care. Which instructions should the nurse provide to the client? Select all that apply.

❑ **1** Wear knee-high hose to prevent edema.

❑ **2** Soak and wash the feet daily using cool water.

❑ **3** Use commercial removers for corns or calluses.

❑ **4** Use over-the-counter preparations to treat ingrown nails.

❑ **5** Apply lanolin or baby oil if dryness is noted along the feet.

❑ **6** Pat the feet dry thoroughly after washing, and dry well between toes.

Answer: 5, 6

Rationale: The nurse should offer the following guidelines in a general hygienic foot and nail care program: inspect the feet daily, including the tops and soles of the feet, the heels, and the areas between the toes; wash the feet daily using lukewarm water, and do not soak the feet; thoroughly pat the feet dry, and dry well between toes; and do not cut corns or calluses or use commercial removers (consult a physician or podiatrist for these problems). Additional general hygienic measures include gently rubbing lanolin, baby oil, or corn oil into the skin if dryness is noted along the feet or between the toes; filing the toe nails straight across and square (do not use scissors or clippers); avoiding the use of over-the-counter preparations to treat ingrown toenails and consulting a physician or podiatrist for these problems; and avoiding wearing elastic stockings, knee-high hose, or constricting garters.

Test-Taking Strategy: Focus on the subject, general hygienic measures for foot and nail care. Eliminate option 1, recalling that constricting items need to be avoided. Eliminate option 2 because of the words *soak* and *cool*. Eliminate options 3 and 4 because of the words *commercial removers* and *over-the-counter,* respectively. Review general hygienic measures for foot and nail care if you had difficulty with this question.

Level of Cognitive Ability: Application
Client Needs: Physiological Integrity
Integrated Process: Teaching and Learning
Content Area: Basic Care and Comfort

Reference

Potter P, Perry A: *Fundamentals of nursing,* ed 6, St Louis, 2005, Mosby, p 1039.

Multiple Response

110. A nurse is assessing a client who is being treated with a beta-adrenergic blocker. Which assessment findings would indicate that the client may be experiencing dose-related side effects of the medication? Select all that apply.

❑ 1 Dizziness
❑ 2 Insomnia
❑ 3 Bradycardia
❑ 4 Reflex tachycardia
❑ 5 Sexual dysfunction
❑ 6 Cardiac dysrhythmias

Answer: 1, 2, 3, 5

Rationale: Beta-adrenergic blockers, commonly called beta-blockers, are useful in treating cardiac dysrhythmias, mild hypertension, mild tachycardia, and angina pectoris. Side effects commonly associated with beta-blockers are usually dose related and include bradycardia, dizziness (hypotensive effect), hypotension, insomnia, and sexual dysfunction (impotence). Options 4 and 6 are reasons for prescribing a beta-blocker; however, these are general side effects of alpha-adrenergic blockers.

Test-Taking Strategy: Specific knowledge regarding the side effects of beta-blockers is needed to select the correct options. However, if you can remember that beta-blockers are useful in treating cardiac dysrhythmias, mild hypertension, mild tachycardia, and angina pectoris, you will be able to eliminate the incorrect options. Review the side effects of this medication classification if you had difficulty with this question.

Level of Cognitive Ability: Analysis
Client Needs: Physiological Integrity
Integrated Process: Nursing Process/Assessment
Content Area: Pharmacological and Parenteral Therapies

Reference
Kee J, Hayes E: *Pharmacology: a nursing process approach,* ed 5, St Louis, 2006, Mosby, pp 274-275.

Multiple Response

111. Atropine sulfate has been prescribed for a client with a hypermotility disorder of the lower urinary tract. The nurse reviews the client's medical record for documentation of which conditions that are contraindicated in the use of this medication? Select all that apply.

❑ **1** Paralytic ileus
❑ **2** Ulcerative colitis
❑ **3** Sinus bradycardia
❑ **4** Narrow-angle glaucoma
❑ **5** Benign prostatic hypertrophy
❑ **6** Obstructive gastrointestinal (GI) disorder

Answer: 1, 2, 4, 5, 6

Rationale: Atropine sulfate is an anticholinergic that inhibits the action of acetylcholine, decreases GI motility and secretory activity, and decreases genitourinary muscle tone. Atropine sulfate and atropine-like drugs (anticholinergic medications) are contraindicated if the client has narrow-angle glaucoma because it can increase intraocular pressure or if the client has paralytic ileus, ulcerative colitis, obstructive GI disorder, intestinal atony, benign prostatic hypertrophy, or myasthenia gravis. It is used to treat sinus bradycardia.

Test-Taking Strategy: Specific knowledge regarding the contraindications to atropine sulfate is needed to select the correct options. However, if you can remember the therapeutic effect of atropine sulfate and that it is an anticholinergic, you will be able to eliminate the incorrect options. Review the contraindications of anticholinergics if you had difficulty with this question.

Level of Cognitive Ability: Analysis
Client Needs: Physiological Integrity
Integrated Process: Nursing Process/Analysis
Content Area: Pharmacological and Parenteral Therapies

References

Hodgson B, Kizior R: *Saunders nursing drug handbook 2007*, Philadelphia, 2007, Saunders, p 103.
Kee J, Hayes E: *Pharmacology: a nursing process approach*, ed 5, St Louis, 2006, Mosby, p 288.

Multiple Response

112. The emergency department nurse is assessing a client who abruptly discontinued benzodiazepine therapy and is experiencing withdrawal symptoms. Which symptoms of withdrawal would the nurse expect to note? Select all that apply.

    ❏ 1 Tremors
    ❏ 2 Sweating
    ❏ 3 Agitation
    ❏ 4 Lethargy
    ❏ 5 Nervousness
    ❏ 6 Muscle weakness

Answer: 1, 2, 3, 5

Rationale: Benzodiazepines should not be abruptly discontinued because withdrawal symptoms are likely to occur. Withdrawal symptoms include agitation, nervousness, insomnia, tremor, anorexia, muscular cramps, and sweating. Withdrawal symptoms from long-term, high-dose benzodiazepine therapy include paranoia, delirium, panic, hypertension, and status epilepticus.

Test-Taking Strategy: Specific knowledge regarding the withdrawal symptoms of benzodiazepines is needed to select the correct options. However, if you can remember that the therapeutic effect of benzodiazepines is anxiolytic, you will be able to eliminate the incorrect options because abrupt withdrawal will produce the opposite effect of an anxiolytic. Review the withdrawal symptoms of benzodiazepines if you had difficulty with this question.

Level of Cognitive Ability: Analysis
Client Needs: Physiological Integrity
Integrated Process: Nursing Process/Assessment
Content Area: Pharmacological and Parenteral Therapies

Reference
Kee J, Hayes E: *Pharmacology: a nursing process approach,* ed 5, St Louis, 2006, Mosby, p 386.

Multiple Response

113. The nurse is caring for a client who is 33 weeks' pregnant and has preterm premature rupture of the membranes (PPROM). Which of the following would the nurse expect to be part of the care plan? Select all that apply.

❑ **1** Monitor for elevated serum creatinine.
❑ **2** Perform frequent biophysical profiles.
❑ **3** Monitor for manifestations of infection.
❑ **4** Teach the client how to count fetal movements.
❑ **5** Use strict sterile technique for vaginal examinations.
❑ **6** Inform the client about the need for tocolytic therapy.

Answer: 2, 3, 4, 5

Rationale: PPROM is membrane rupture before 37 weeks of gestation. Whenever PPROM is suspected, strict sterile technique should be used in any vaginal examination to prevent infection. Frequent biophysical profiles are performed to determine fetal health status and estimate amniotic fluid volume. Monitoring for signs of infection is a major part of the nursing care. The woman should also be taught how to count fetal movements daily, since slowing of fetal movement has been shown to be a precursor to severe fetal compromise. Elevated serum creatinine does not occur in PPROM but may be noted in severe preeclampsia. Tocolytic therapy is used for women in preterm labor (not for PPROM).

Test-Taking Strategy: Focus on the client's condition, PPROM, and think about the pathophysiology of this condition. Select options 3 and 5 because they relate to preventing infection. Next select options 2 and 4 because they relate to determining fetal health status. Recalling the causes of an elevated serum creatinine and the purpose of tocolytic therapy will assist in eliminating these options. Review the care plan for a client with PPROM if you had difficulty with this question.

Level of Cognitive Ability: Analysis
Client Needs: Physiological Integrity
Integrated Process: Nursing Process/Planning
Content Area: Physiological Adaptation

Reference
Wong D, Perry S, Hockenberry M, et al: *Maternal child nursing care,* ed 3, St Louis, 2006, Mosby, p 554.

Multiple Response

114. What clinical manifestations would the nurse expect to find in a client who has superficial thrombophlebitis. Select all that apply.

- ❏ **1** Redness noted along the vein
- ❏ **2** Induration noted along the vein
- ❏ **3** Warmth palpated along the vein
- ❏ **4** Tenderness on palpation of the vein
- ❏ **5** Diminished pulses in the affected extremity
- ❏ **6** Dilated blue-colored veins noted along the length of the extremity

Answer: 1, 2, 3, 4

Rationale: Superficial thrombophlebitis is an inflammation of a superficial vein accompanied by the formation of a clot. Clinical manifestations of superficial thrombophlebitis include redness (rubor), induration, warmth (calor), and tenderness (dolor) along a vein. Discomfort may be relieved by applying heat. Activity is encouraged as prescribed, and a supportive wrap or stocking should be applied. Diminished pulses and dilated blue-colored veins are not manifestations of superficial thrombophlebitis.

Test-Taking Strategy: Focus on the subject, superficial thrombophlebitis. Remember that the suffix *-itis* indicates an inflammation. This will assist in eliminating option 6. Next, recalling that this disorder involves a vein, not an artery, will assist in eliminating option 5. Review the manifestations of superficial thrombophlebitis if you had difficulty with this question.

Level of Cognitive Ability: Analysis
Client Needs: Physiological Integrity
Integrated Process: Nursing Process/Assessment
Content Area: Physiological Adaptation

Reference
Black J, Hawks J: *Medical-surgical nursing: clinical management for positive outcomes,* ed 7, Philadelphia, 2005, Saunders, p 1537.

Multiple Response

115. In caring for a client with myasthenia gravis, the nurse should be alert for which of the following manifestations of myasthenic crisis? Select all that apply.

1 ❑ Bradycardia
2 ❑ Increased diaphoresis
3 ❑ Decreased lacrimation
4 ❑ Bowel and bladder incontinence
5 ❑ Absent cough and swallow reflex
6 ❑ Sudden marked rise in blood pressure

Answer: 2, 4, 5, 6

Rationale: Myasthenic crisis is caused by undermedication or can be precipitated by an infection or sudden withdrawal of anticholinesterase drugs. It may also occur spontaneously. Clinical manifestations include sudden marked rise in blood pressure because of hypoxia; increased heart rate; severe respiratory distress and cyanosis; absent cough and swallow reflex; increased secretions, increased diaphoresis, and increased lacrimation; restlessness; dysarthria; and bowel and bladder incontinence.

Test-Taking Strategy: Specific knowledge regarding the manifestations of myasthenic crisis is needed to answer this question. Recall that myasthenic crisis is caused by undermedication. With this in mind, think about the manifestations of myasthenia gravis to assist in selecting the correct options. Review the manifestations of myasthenic crisis if you had difficulty with this question.

Level of Cognitive Ability: Analysis
Client Needs: Physiological Integrity
Integrated Process: Nursing Process/Assessment
Content Area: Physiological Adaptation

Reference

Black J, Hawks J: *Medical-surgical nursing: clinical management for positive outcomes,* ed 7, Philadelphia, 2005, Saunders, p 2184.

Multiple Response

116. A client taking diuretics is at risk for hypokalemia. The nurse monitors for which of the following clinical manifestations of hypokalemia? Select all that apply.

❏ **1** Muscle twitches
❏ **2** Tall T waves on electrocardiogram (ECG)
❏ **3** Deep tendon hyporeflexia
❏ **4** General skeletal muscle weakness
❏ **5** Hypoactive to absent bowel sounds
❏ **6** Prominent U wave on ECG

Answer: 3, 4, 5, 6

Rationale: Hypokalemia is a serum potassium level below 3.5 mEq/L. Clinical manifestations include ECG abnormalities such as ST depression, inverted T wave, prominent U wave, and heart block. Other manifestations include shallow ineffective respirations and diminished breath sounds; general skeletal muscle weakness and deep tendon hyporeflexia; decreased bowel motility and hypoactive to absent bowel sounds; and polyuria, decreased ability to concentrate urine, and decreased urine specific gravity. Tall T waves and muscle twitches are manifestations of hyperkalemia.

Test-Taking Strategy: Focus on the subject, the manifestations of hypokalemia. Note that options 3, 4, and 5 are comparative or alike in that they identify a decreased, or *hypo-*, response; these are manifestations of *hypo*kalemia. Next remember that a prominent U wave on ECG is a manifestation of hypokalemia. Review the manifestations of hypokalemia if you had difficulty with this question.

Level of Cognitive Ability: Analysis
Client Needs: Physiological Integrity
Integrated Process: Nursing Process/Assessment
Content Area: Physiological Adaptation

Reference
Ignatavicius D, Workman M: *Medical surgical nursing: critical thinking for collaborative care,* ed 5, Philadelphia, 2006, Saunders, p 228.

Multiple Response

117. The nurse provides dietary instructions to a client who needs to limit intake of sodium. The nurse instructs the client that which food items need to be avoided because of their high-sodium content? Select all that apply.

❑ 1 Apples
❑ 2 Broccoli
❑ 3 Soy sauce
❑ 4 Asparagus
❑ 5 Cantaloupe
❑ 6 Cured pork

Answer: 3, 6

Rationale: Foods highest in sodium include table salt, some cheeses, soy sauce, cured pork, canned foods because of the preservatives, and foods such as cold cuts. Fruits and vegetables contain minimal amounts of sodium.

Test-Taking Strategy: Focus on the subject, foods high in sodium. Eliminate options 1, 2, 4, and 5 because they are comparative or alike in that they are fruits and vegetables and are low in sodium. Review high-sodium foods if you had difficulty with this question.

Level of Cognitive Ability: Application
Client Needs: Physiological Integrity
Integrated Process: Teaching and Learning
Content Area: Reduction of Risk Potential

Reference
Ignatavicius D, Workman M: *Medical surgical nursing: critical thinking for collaborative care,* ed 5, Philadelphia, 2006, Saunders, p 205.

Multiple Response

118. The nurse prepares a list of home care instructions for a client following total hip replacement. Which instructions should the nurse place on the list? Select all that apply.

❑ 1 Sit with the legs elevated as much as possible.

❑ 2 Use assistive devices for putting on shoes and socks.

❑ 3 Avoid crossing the legs beyond the midline of the body.

❑ 4 Contact the surgeon if drainage occurs from the incision.

❑ 5 Cleanse the hip incision with a mild soap and water daily.

❑ 6 Expect consistent increased hip pain as mobility increases.

Answer: 2, 3, 4, 5

Rationale: After total hip replacement, measures are taken to avoid dislocation and to prevent other postoperative complications such as infection. The client is instructed not to bend the hip more than 90 degrees and to avoid sitting or standing for prolonged periods. The client should not cross the legs beyond the midline of the body and should use assistive or adaptive devices to assist in dressing. The client is taught to inspect the incision daily; to cleanse the hip incision with a mild soap and water daily; and to report any redness, heat, or drainage to the surgeon immediately. Although some postoperative pain is expected, consistent increased hip pain is not expected.

Test-Taking Strategy: Focus on the subject, instructions for a client after total hip replacement. Recalling the signs of infection and that measures are taken to avoid dislocation will assist in answering correctly. Review home care instructions for a client after total hip replacement if you had difficulty with this question.

Level of Cognitive Ability: Application
Client Needs: Physiological Integrity
Integrated Process: Teaching and Learning
Content Area: Reduction of Risk Potential

Reference
Ignatavicius D, Workman M: *Medical surgical nursing: critical thinking for collaborative care,* ed 5, Philadelphia, 2006, Saunders, p 389.

Multiple Response

119. The nurse provides which instructions to the client about the prevention and early detection of Lyme disease? Select all that apply.

❏ **1** Wear dark clothing when walking in wooded areas.

❏ **2** Avoid heavily wooded areas and areas with thick underbrush.

❏ **3** Wear long-sleeved tops and long pants with closed shoes and a hat or cap.

❏ **4** Bathe after being in an infested area, and inspect the body carefully for ticks.

❏ **5** Avoid the use of insect repellent on the skin and clothing because of its toxicity.

❏ **6** If a tick is found, report to the physician immediately for a blood test to detect the presence of Lyme disease.

Answer: 2, 3, 4

Rationale: Lyme disease is a systemic infectious disease caused by the spirochete *Borrelia burgdorferi* and results from the bite of an infected deer tick. Client instructions for the prevention and early detection of Lyme disease include avoid heavily wooded areas and areas with thick underbrush, walk in the center of trails in wooded areas, avoid wearing dark clothing because lighter colored clothing makes spotting ticks easier, use insect repellent on the skin and clothing when in an area where ticks are likely to be found, wear long-sleeved tops and long pants with closed shoes and a hat or cap, bathe immediately after being in an infested area and inspect the body carefully for ticks, gently remove a tick from the skin with tweezers and flush it down the toilet, and report flulike symptoms to the physician. Lyme disease blood testing is not reliable until 4 to 6 weeks after being bitten by the tick.

Test-Taking Strategy: Focus on the subject, prevention and early detection of Lyme disease. Recalling that Lyme disease results from the bite of an infected deer tick will assist in selecting options 2, 3, and 4. Next, eliminate option 1 because of the words *dark clothing* and option 6 because of the word *immediately.* Also remember that Lyme disease blood testing is not reliable until 4 to 6 weeks after being bitten by the tick. Review these measures if you had difficulty with this question.

Level of Cognitive Ability: Application
Client Needs: Physiological Integrity
Integrated Process: Teaching and Learning
Content Area: Reduction of Risk Potential

Reference
Ignatavicius D, Workman M: *Medical surgical nursing: critical thinking for collaborative care,* ed 5, Philadelphia, 2006, Saunders, p 418.

Multiple Response

120. A nurse is caring for a client who is at risk for a pressure ulcer. Which of the following interventions should be included in the care plan to prevent a pressure ulcer? Select all that apply.

❑ **1** Minimize the force and friction applied to the skin.

❑ **2** Perform a systematic skin inspection at least once a day.

❑ **3** Massage vigorously over bony prominences twice daily.

❑ **4** Cleanse the skin at the time of soiling and at routine intervals.

❑ **5** Use pillows to keep the knees and other bony prominences from direct contact with one another.

❑ **6** Use hot water and a mild cleansing agent that minimizes irritation and dryness of the skin when bathing the client.

Answer: 1, 2, 4, 5

Rationale: Interventions for prevention of pressure ulcers include performing a systematic skin inspection at least once a day, giving particular attention to the bony prominences; cleansing the skin at the time of soiling and at routine intervals; avoiding the use of hot water; using a mild cleansing agent that minimizes irritation and dryness of the skin; and minimizing the force and friction applied to the skin. Pillows should be used to keep the knees and other bony prominences from direct contact with one another, since skin contact can promote breakdown. Massaging over bony prominences (especially vigorous) can be harmful to at-risk skin surfaces.

Test-Taking Strategy: Focus on the subject, preventing a pressure ulcer. Visualize each of the options in terms of how it will prevent or promote skin breakdown. Eliminate option 3 because of the word *vigorously* and option 6 because of the word *hot.* Review measures to prevent a pressure ulcer if you had difficulty with this question.

Level of Cognitive Ability: Application
Client Needs: Physiological Integrity
Integrated Process: Nursing Process/Planning
Content Area: Reduction of Risk Potential

Reference
Black J, Hawks J: *Medical-surgical nursing: clinical management for positive outcomes,* ed 7, Philadelphia, 2005, Saunders, p 1408.

Multiple Response

121. A client is diagnosed with Goodpasture's syndrome. The nurse expects to note which clinical manifestations on assessment of the client? Select all that apply.

- ❏ 1 Weight loss
- ❏ 2 Hemoptysis
- ❏ 3 Hypertension
- ❏ 4 Shortness of breath
- ❏ 5 Increased urinary output
- ❏ 6 Generalized nondependent edema

Answer: 2, 3, 4, 6

Rationale: Goodpasture's syndrome is an autoimmune disorder in which autoantibodies are made against the glomerular basement membrane and neutrophils. The two organs primarily affected are the lungs and kidneys. Lung damage manifests as pulmonary hemorrhage. Kidney damage manifests as glomerulonephritis that may rapidly progress to complete kidney failure. Manifestations include shortness of breath, hemoptysis, decreased urinary output, weight gain, generalized nondependent edema, hypertension, and tachycardia.

Test-Taking Strategy: Focus on the client's diagnosis and recall that the two organs primarily affected in this disorder are the lungs and kidneys. This will assist in eliminating options 1 and 5, since weight gain and decreased urinary output are more likely to occur in a kidney disorder. Review the manifestations of Goodpasture's syndrome if you had difficulty with this question.

Level of Cognitive Ability: Analysis
Client Needs: Physiological Integrity
Integrated Process: Nursing Process/Assessment
Content Area: Physiological Adaptation

Reference
Ignatavicius D, Workman M: *Medical surgical nursing: critical thinking for collaborative care,* ed 5, Philadelphia, 2006, Saunders, p 464.

Multiple Response

122. A nurse monitors a client with a tumor of the esophagus for signs of superior vena cava (SVC) syndrome. Which of the following are signs of this complication? Select all that apply.

- ❑ 1 Nosebleeds
- ❑ 2 Edema in the eyes
- ❑ 3 Edema in the hands
- ❑ 4 Difficulty breathing
- ❑ 5 Mental status changes
- ❑ 6 Weight loss with complaints of looseness of clothing, especially around the neck

Answer: 1, 2, 3, 4, 5

Rationale: SVC syndrome occurs when the SVC is compressed or obstructed by tumor growth. The manifestations result from the blockage of blood flow in the venous system of the head, neck, and upper trunk. Early manifestations occur when the client arises after a night's sleep and include edema of the face, especially around the eyes, and tightness of the shirt or blouse collar (Stokes' sign). As the compression worsens, edema in the hands and arms, dyspnea, erythema of the upper body, and epistaxis occur. Late manifestations include hemorrhage, cyanosis, mental status changes, decreased cardiac output, and hypotension.

Test-Taking Strategy: Recall that SVC syndrome is caused by a compression or obstruction by tumor growth and that manifestations result from the blockage of blood flow in the venous system of the head, neck, and upper trunk. With this in mind, read each option and determine how it relates to this pathophysiology. The only option that does not correlate with this pathophysiology is option 6. Review the manifestations of SVC syndrome if you had difficulty with this question.

Level of Cognitive Ability: Analysis
Client Needs: Physiological Integrity
Integrated Process: Nursing Process/Assessment
Content Area: Physiological Adaptation

Reference
Ignatavicius D, Workman M: *Medical surgical nursing: critical thinking for collaborative care,* ed 5, Philadelphia, 2006, Saunders, pp 502-503.

Multiple Response

123. What equipment should be kept at the bedside of a client who has a tracheostomy tube? Select all that apply.

- ❑ **1** Scissors
- ❑ **2** Obturator
- ❑ **3** Suture set
- ❑ **4** Resuscitation bag
- ❑ **5** Tracheal dilator (spreaders)
- ❑ **6** Extra tracheostomy tube of the same size

Answer: 2, 4, 5, 6

Rationale: A tracheostomy is the surgical creation of a stoma, or opening, into the trachea through the underlying skin. The following equipment should be kept at the client's bedside: extra tracheostomy tube of the same size and one size smaller, obturator belonging to the existing tube, tracheal dilator (spreaders), oxygen source, suction catheters and suction source, and a resuscitation bag. This equipment needs to be available in the event of accidental decannulation. Scissors and a suture set are unnecessary.

Test-Taking Strategy: Focus on the subject, equipment to be kept at the bedside of a client who has a tracheostomy tube. Use the ABCs, airway, breathing, and circulation, to direct you to the correct options. Review care of the client with a tracheostomy tube if you had difficulty with this question.

Level of Cognitive Ability: Application
Client Needs: Physiological Integrity
Integrated Process: Nursing Process/Implementation
Content Area: Reduction of Risk Potential

Reference
Black J, Hawks J: *Medical-surgical nursing: clinical management for positive outcomes,* ed 7, Philadelphia, 2005, Saunders, p 1780.

Multiple Response

124. A nurse is assessing a client who has a thoracic (T-10) spinal cord injury. Which assessments are specific to this level of spinal cord involvement? Select all that apply.

- ❏ **1** Bowel and bladder function
- ❏ **2** Reflexes in the lower extremities
- ❏ **3** Pain sensation in the upper extremities
- ❏ **4** Sensory function of the upper extremities
- ❏ **5** Voluntary movement of the lower extremities
- ❏ **6** Ability to take breaths independent of a ventilator

Answer: 1, 2, 5

Rationale: Below the level of spinal cord injury, the client loses voluntary movement; sensation of pain, temperature, pressure, and proprioception; bowel and bladder function; and spinal and autonomic reflexes. A client with a thoracic (T-10) spinal cord injury will have the loss of function in the lower extremities, including problems with bowel and bladder function. A client with a cervical spinal cord injury will experience problems with breathing.

Test-Taking Strategy: Focus on the client's level of spinal cord injury. Visualizing the position of a T-10 injury will assist in eliminating options 3, 4, and 6 because they are functions that take place above the client's level of injury. Review assessment of a client with a spinal cord injury if you had difficulty with this question.

Level of Cognitive Ability: Analysis
Client Needs: Physiological Integrity
Integrated Process: Nursing Process/Assessment
Content Area: Physiological Adaptation

Reference
Black J, Hawks J: *Medical-surgical nursing: clinical management for positive outcomes,* ed 7, Philadelphia, 2005, Saunders, pp 2024, 2214.

Figure/Illustration with a Multiple Choice

125. The nurse performs client rounds and notes that a client with a respiratory disorder is wearing this oxygen device. (Refer to figure.) The nurse documents that the client is receiving oxygen by which type of low-flow oxygen delivery system?

❏ **1** Venturi mask
❏ **2** Nasal cannula
❏ **3** Simple face mask
❏ **4** Partial rebreather mask

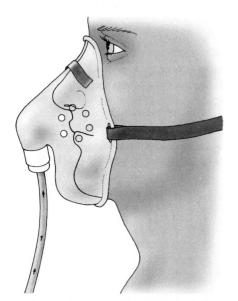

From Ignatavicius D, Workman M: *Medical surgical nursing: critical thinking for collaborative care,* ed 5, Philadelphia, 2006, Saunders.

Answer: 3

Rationale: A simple face mask is used to deliver oxygen concentrations of 40% to 60% for short-term oxygen therapy or in an emergency. A minimum flow rate of 5 L/min is needed to prevent the rebreathing of exhaled air. The simple face mask fits over the nose and mouth, has exhalation ports, and has a tube that connects to the oxygen source. A Venturi mask is a high-flow oxygen delivery system that delivers the most accurate oxygen concentration. An adaptor is located between the bottom of the mask and the oxygen source. The adaptor contains holes of different sizes that allow specific amounts of air to mix with the oxygen. The nasal cannula contains nasal prongs that are used to deliver oxygen flow rates at 1 to 6 L/min. A partial rebreather mask is a mask with a reservoir bag without flaps. It provides oxygen concentrations of 60% to 75% with flow rates of 6 to 11 L/min.

Test-Taking Strategy: Note the type of mask in the figure/illustration. Note that it simply illustrates an oxygen mask fitted over the client's nose and mouth. This will assist in answering correctly. Re-view the various types of oxygen delivery systems if you had difficulty with this question.

Level of Cognitive Ability: Analysis
Client Needs: Physiological Integrity
Integrated Process: Communication and Documentation
Content Area: Reduction of Risk Potential

Reference

Ignatavicius D, Workman M: *Medical surgical nursing: critical thinking for collaborative care,* ed 5, Philadelphia, 2006, Saunders, pp 548-550.

Multiple Response

126. A client is suspected of having deep venous thrombosis (DVT). The nurse anticipates that which diagnostic studies will be prescribed to assist in the diagnosis of this disorder? Select all that apply.

❑ **1** Platelet count
❑ **2** D-dimer blood test
❑ **3** Electrocardiography
❑ **4** Venous duplex scanning
❑ **5** Magnetic resonance imaging (MRI)
❑ **6** International normalized ratio (INR)

Answer: 2, 4

Rationale: DVT is a disorder involving a thrombus in one of the deep veins of the body, most commonly the iliac or femoral veins. Venous duplex scanning is a primary diagnostic test for DVT because it allows visualization of the vein, which provides a reliable diagnosis of venous thrombus. The D-dimer blood test is also used in evaluation of DVT. The D dimer is a product of fibrin degradation and is indicative of fibrinolysis, which occurs with thrombosis. A platelet count will not provide information related to the presence of DVT. An INR is a blood test used to evaluate the effectiveness of warfarin (Coumadin) therapy. Electrocardiography evaluates the electrical activity of the heart. An MRI may be used for a variety of reasons, such as to detect the presence of a tumor. It will not diagnose DVT.

Test-Taking Strategy: Focus on the subject, diagnostic studies for DVT. Think about the pathophysiology associated with DVT, and think about each test in the options and how it may or may not relate to this pathophysiology. This will direct you to the correct options. Review diagnostic studies for DVT if you had difficulty with this question.

Level of Cognitive Ability: Analysis
Client Needs: Physiological Integrity
Integrated Process: Nursing Process/Analysis
Content Area: Physiological Adaptation

Reference
Black J, Hawks J: *Medical-surgical nursing: clinical management for positive outcomes,* ed 7, Philadelphia, 2005, Saunders, p 1537.

Multiple Response

127. The nurse is assessing the function of a Pleur-evac chest drainage system attached to a client who had a thoracotomy 1 day ago. The nurse expects to note which of the following? Select all that apply.

❑ **1** Drainage of 50 mL/hr
❑ **2** Pink fluid in the drainage collection chamber
❑ **3** Excessive bubbling in the water seal chamber
❑ **4** Gentle bubbling in the suction control chamber
❑ **5** Fluctuation of fluid in the tube in the water seal chamber
❑ **6** The chest drainage tubing resting on the bed under the client's legs

Answer: 1, 2, 4, 5

Rationale: The Pleur-evac chest drainage system is a device using a one-piece disposable plastic unit with three chambers (drainage, water seal, suction control) that duplicates the three-bottle system. The drainage collection chamber collects drainage from the client's pleural space. An amount of 50 mL/hr is not excessive in a 1-day postoperative client; however, the physician is notified if drainage of more than 100 mL/hr occurs. The water seal chamber prevents water from entering the pleural space. Bubbling in this chamber indicates air drainage from the client. Excessive bubbling may indicate an air leak in the system; if this occurs, further intervention is needed to locate the air leak. Fluctuation of fluid in the tube in the water seal chamber is expected and occurs as the client inhales and exhales. Gentle bubbling should be noted in the suction control chamber when suction is applied. The chest drainage tubing should not be kinked or obstructed (e.g., from the client lying on the tube) because this will build pressure in the system, disrupt its functioning, and harm the client.

Test-Taking Strategy: Think about the purpose of the chest drainage system and each chamber of the system. Read each option keeping this in mind, and note that the client is 1 day postoperative. Eliminate option 3 because of the word *excessive* and option 6 because of the words *under the client's legs*. Review care to the client with a chest tube drainage system if you had difficulty with this question.

Level of Cognitive Ability: Analysis
Client Needs: Physiological Integrity
Integrated Process: Nursing Process/Evaluation
Content Area: Reduction of Risk Potential

Reference
Black J, Hawks J: *Medical-surgical nursing: clinical management for positive outcomes,* ed 7, Philadelphia, 2005, Saunders, pp 623-624.

Figure/Illustration with a Fill-in-the-Blank

128. The nurse hangs an intravenous (IV) bag of 1000 mL of 5% dextrose in water (D_5W) at 3 PM and sets the flow rate to infuse at 75 mL/hr. At 11 PM, the nurse would expect the fluid remaining in the IV bag to be at approximately which level? (Refer to figure.)

Answer: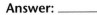

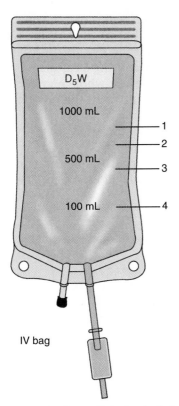

IV bag

From Kee J, Marshall S: *Clinical calculations: with applications to general and specialty areas,* ed 5, Philadelphia, 2004, Saunders.

Answer: 3

Rationale: In an 8-hour period, 600 mL would infuse if an IV is set to infuse at 75 mL/hr. Therefore 400 mL would remain in the IV bag.

Test-Taking Strategy: Focus on the data in the question and use simple math to determine that in an 8-hour period (3 to 11 PM), 600 mL would infuse (8 hr × 75 mL/hr = 600 mL). This means that 400 mL would remain. Perform the calculation and then verify your answer using a calculator. Review calculations related to IV infusions if you had difficulty with this question.

Level of Cognitive Ability: Analysis
Client Needs: Physiological Integrity
Integrated Process: Nursing Process/Assessment
Content Area: Pharmacological and Parenteral Therapies

Reference
Kee J, Marshall S: *Clinical calculations: with applications to general and specialty areas,* ed 5, Philadelphia, 2004, Saunders, p 202.

Fill-in-the-Blank

129. A physician orders 1000 mL of normal saline to infuse at 100 mL/hr. The drop factor is 10 drops/mL. The nurse sets the flow rate at how many drops per minute? (Round answer to the nearest whole number.)

Answer: _____ drops/min

Answer: 17

Rationale: It will take 10 hours for 1000 mL to infuse at 100 mL/hr (1000 mL ÷ 100 mL = 10 hr). Next, use the intravenous (IV) flow rate formula.

Formula

$$\frac{\text{Total volume} \times \text{Drop factor}}{\text{Time in minutes}} = \text{Drops/min}$$

$$\frac{1000 \text{ mL} \times 10 \text{ drops/mL}}{600 \text{ min}} = \frac{10{,}000}{600} = 16.6, \text{ or } 17 \text{ drops/min}$$

Test-Taking Strategy: Focus on the data in the question. First, determine how many hours that it will take for 1000 mL to infuse at 100 mL/hr. Next use the formula for calculating IV flow rates and verify the answer using a calculator. Remember to round the answer to the nearest whole number. Review IV infusion rates if you had difficulty with this question.

Level of Cognitive Ability: Application
Client Needs: Physiological Integrity
Integrated Process: Nursing Process/Implementation
Content Area: Pharmacological and Parenteral Therapies

Reference
Kee J, Marshall S: *Clinical calculations: with applications to general and specialty areas,* ed 5, Philadelphia, 2004, Saunders, p 212.

Multiple Response

130. A nurse is performing an assessment on a client who has chronic venous insufficiency. Which of the following clinical manifestations would the nurse expect the client to exhibit? Select all that apply.

❑ **1** Intermittent claudication
❑ **2** Brown discoloration of the skin
❑ **3** Dry and flaky skin and complaints of itching
❑ **4** Edema that worsens at the end of the day
❑ **5** Complaints of aching and heaviness in the legs
❑ **6** Decreased or absence of arterial pulses in the affected extremity

Answer: 2, 3, 4, 5

Rationale: Venous insufficiency is an abnormal circulatory condition characterized by decreased return of venous blood from the legs to the trunk of the body. The client who has venous disease may report chronic aching pain and heaviness in the legs when they are in a dependent position. Additional manifestations include edema that worsens at the end of the day, dry and flaky skin and complaints of itching, brown discoloration of the skin, and dependent cyanosis. Skin temperature remains normal or may be slightly warmer than the unaffected area, and pulses are present, although they may be difficult to palpate if edema is present. Intermittent claudication and decreased or absent pulses are characteristics of arterial insufficiency.

Test-Taking Strategy: Focus on the subject, the manifestations of chronic venous insufficiency. The strategic word in this question is *venous.* Think about the anatomy and physiology of the venous system to assist in answering the question. Remember that intermittent claudication and decreased or absent pulses are characteristics of arterial, not venous, insufficiency. Review the manifestations of both arterial and venous insufficiency if you had difficulty with this question.

Level of Cognitive Ability: Analysis
Client Needs: Physiological Integrity
Integrated Process: Nursing Process/Assessment
Content Area: Physiological Adaptation

References
Black J, Hawks J: *Medical-surgical nursing: clinical management for positive outcomes,* ed 7, Philadelphia, 2005, Saunders, pp 1477-1478.
Mosby's medical, nursing, and allied health dictionary, ed 7, St Louis, 2006, Mosby, p 1949.

Multiple Response

131. The nurse is caring for a client receiving digoxin (Lanoxin). Which of the following manifestations correlate with a digoxin level of 2.3 ng/dL? Select all that apply.

❏ **1** Nausea
❏ **2** Drowsiness
❏ **3** Photophobia
❏ **4** Increased appetite
❏ **5** Increased energy level
❏ **6** Seeing halos around bright objects

Answer: 1, 2, 3, 6

Rationale: Digoxin is a cardiac glycoside used to manage and treat heart failure, control ventricular rate in clients with atrial fibrillation, and treat and prevent recurrent paroxysmal atrial tachycardia. The therapeutic range is 0.8 to 2.0 ng/dL. Signs of toxicity include gastrointestinal disturbances, including anorexia, nausea, and vomiting; neurological abnormalities such as fatigue, headache, depression, weakness, drowsiness, confusion, and nightmares; facial pain; personality changes; and ocular disturbances such as photophobia, halos around bright lights, and yellow or green color perception.

Test-Taking Strategy: Note the strategic words *2.3 ng/dL.* Recalling that signs of digoxin toxicity include gastrointestinal disturbances, neurological abnormalities, and ocular disturbances will assist in answering the question correctly. Review this therapeutic range and the signs of digoxin toxicity if you had difficulty with this question.

Level of Cognitive Ability: Analysis
Client Needs: Physiological Integrity
Integrated Process: Nursing Process/Assessment
Content Area: Pharmacological and Parenteral Therapies

Reference
Hodgson B, Kizior R: *Saunders nursing drug handbook 2007,* Philadelphia, 2007, Saunders, p 357.

Multiple Response

132. The emergency department nurse prepares for which interventions in the care of a child with epiglottitis? Select all that apply.

- ❏ **1** Obtaining a chest x-ray
- ❏ **2** Obtaining a throat culture
- ❏ **3** Monitoring pulse oximetry
- ❏ **4** Maintaining a patent airway
- ❏ **5** Providing humidified oxygen
- ❏ **6** Administering antipyretics and antibiotics

Answer: 1, 3, 4, 5, 6

Rationale: Epiglottitis is an acute inflammation and swelling of the epiglottis and surrounding tissue. It is a life-threatening, rapidly progressive condition that may cause complete airway obstruction within a few hours of onset. The most reliable diagnostic sign is an edematous, cherry-red epiglottis. The primary concern is the development of complete airway obstruction. Therefore the child's throat is not examined or cultured because any stimulation with a tongue depressor or culture swab could trigger complete airway obstruction. Some interventions include maintaining a patent airway, providing humidified oxygen, monitoring pulse oximetry, obtaining a chest x-ray film, and administering antipyretics and antibiotics. The child may also require intubation and mechanical ventilation.

Test-Taking Strategy: Recall the pathophysiology associated with epiglottitis. Remember that the primary concern is the development of complete airway obstruction and that any stimulation with a tongue depressor or culture swab could trigger complete airway obstruction. This will assist in eliminating the only incorrect option, option 2. Review interventions in the care of a child with epiglottitis if you had difficulty with this question.

Level of Cognitive Ability: Analysis
Client Needs: Physiological Integrity
Integrated Process: Nursing Process/Implementation
Content Area: Physiological Adaptation

Reference
McKinney E, James S, Murray S, et al: *Maternal-child nursing,* ed 2, Philadelphia, 2005, Saunders, p 1210.

Multiple Response

133. A child with rheumatic fever is admitted to the hospital. The nurse reviews the child's record and expects to note which clinical manifestations documented in the record? Select all that apply.

❑ **1** Cardiac murmur
❑ **2** Cardiac enlargement
❑ **3** Cool pale skin over the joints
❑ **4** White painful skin lesions on the trunk
❑ **5** Small nontender lumps on bony prominences
❑ **6** Purposeless jerky movements of the extremities and face

Answer: 1, 2, 5, 6

Rationale: Rheumatic fever is a systemic inflammatory disease that may develop as a delayed reaction to an inadequately treated infection of the upper respiratory tract by group A beta-hemolytic streptococci. Clinical manifestations of rheumatic fever are related to the inflammatory response. Major manifestations include arthritis manifested as tender, warm erythematous joints; carditis manifested as inflammation of the endocardium, including the valves, myocardium, and pericardium; cardiac murmur and cardiac enlargement; chorea, manifested as involuntary, purposeless jerky movements of the legs, arms, and face with speech impairment; erythema marginatum, manifested as red, painless skin lesions usually over the trunk; and subcutaneous nodules, manifested as small nontender lumps on joints and bony prominences.

Test-Taking Strategy: Note the strategic word *fever*. Recalling that rheumatic fever is a systemic inflammatory disease and noting the words *cool* in option 3 and *white* in option 4 will assist in answering this question. Remember that the client will exhibit tender, warm, erythematous joints and red, painless skin lesions usually over the trunk. Review the clinical manifestations of rheumatic fever if you had difficulty with this question.

Level of Cognitive Ability: Analysis
Client Needs: Physiological Integrity
Integrated Process: Nursing Process/Assessment
Content Area: Physiological Adaptation

Reference
McKinney E, James S, Murray S, et al: *Maternal-child nursing,* ed 2, Philadelphia, 2005, Saunders, p 1287.

Multiple Response

134. A nurse is performing an admission assessment on a client with a diagnosis of heart failure. Which of the following manifestations would indicate to the nurse that the client is experiencing left-sided heart failure? Select all that apply.

- ❏ **1** Dyspnea
- ❏ **2** Dependent edema
- ❏ **3** Crackles in the lungs
- ❏ **4** Frothy pink-tinged sputum
- ❏ **5** Jugular neck vein distention
- ❏ **6** Hacking cough that worsens at night

Answer: 1, 3, 4, 6

Rationale: Heart failure is a condition that refers to the inadequacy of the heart to pump blood throughout the body. The manifestations of left-sided heart failure are respiratory and reflect the pulmonary congestion that occurs. These manifestations include a hacking cough that worsens at night, dyspnea and breathlessness, crackles or wheezes in the lungs, and frothy or pink-tinged sputum. Manifestations of right-sided failure reflect the systemic congestion that occurs. These manifestations include jugular neck vein distention, enlarged liver and spleen, anorexia and nausea, dependent edema, distended abdomen, swollen hands and fingers, polyuria at night, weight gain, and hypertension.

Test-Taking Strategy: Note the subject of the question, manifestations of left-sided heart failure. Remember *"left and lungs"* to assist in determining the manifestations of left-sided heart failure. Remember that right-sided failure affects the systemic circulation. Review the manifestations of left-sided and right-sided heart failure if you had difficulty with this question.

Level of Cognitive Ability: Analysis
Client Needs: Physiological Integrity
Integrated Process: Nursing Process/Assessment
Content Area: Physiological Adaptation

Reference
Ignatavicius D, Workman M: *Medical surgical nursing: critical thinking for collaborative care,* ed 5, Philadelphia, 2006, Saunders, p 753.

Figure/Illustration with a Fill-in-the-Blank

135. The nurse needs to draw 0.6 mL of medication into a syringe. The nurse fills the syringe with medication to which area on the syringe? (Refer to figure.)

Answer: _____

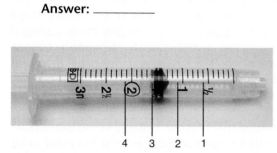

From Macklin D, Chernecky C, Infortuna H: *Math for clinical practice,* St Louis, 2005, Mosby.

Answer: 1

Rationale: The 3-mL syringe is calibrated in tenths (0.1 mL). Therefore, if the nurse needs to draw 0.6 mL, this amount would be located one line (0.1 mL) past the ¹/₂ point.

Test-Taking Strategy: Focus on the figure and note that it illustrates a 3-mL syringe. Recalling that a 3-mL syringe is calibrated in tenths (0.1 mL) will direct you to the correct option. Review medication administration using a 3-mL syringe if you had difficulty with this question.

Level of Cognitive Ability: Application
Client Needs: Physiological Integrity
Integrated Process: Nursing Process/Implementation
Content Area: Pharmacological and Parenteral Therapies

References

Kee J, Marshall S: *Clinical calculations: with applications to general and specialty areas,* ed 5, Philadelphia, 2004, Saunders, p 149.
Macklin D, Chernecky C, Infortuna H: *Math for clinical practice,* St Louis, 2005, Mosby, p 587.

Multiple Response

136. The nurse is assessing a client with a suspected diagnosis of myocardial infarction. Which of the following are characteristics of the substernal chest pain that occurs with this condition? Select all that apply.

❏ **1** Occurs without cause
❏ **2** Lasts 30 minutes or longer
❏ **3** Is relieved only by opioids
❏ **4** Usually occurs in the morning
❏ **5** Is precipitated by exertion or stress
❏ **6** Radiates to the left arm, back, or jaw

Answer: 1, 2, 3, 4, 6

Rationale: Myocardial infarction occurs when myocardial tissue is abruptly and severely deprived of oxygen. The substernal chest pain that occurs in myocardial infarction radiates to the left arm, back, or jaw; occurs without cause, usually in the morning; is relieved only by opioids; and lasts 30 minutes or longer. The client with myocardial infarction also experiences nausea, diaphoresis, dyspnea, dysrhythmias, epigastric distress, and fatigue. Angina is a temporary imbalance between the coronary artery's ability to supply oxygen and the cardiac muscle's demand for oxygen. The substernal chest pain that occurs in angina radiates to the left arm, is precipitated by exertion or stress, is relieved by rest or nitroglycerin, and lasts less than 15 minutes.

Test-Taking Strategy: Focus on the subject, the characteristics of the substernal chest pain that occurs with myocardial infarction. Remember that pain that occurs with myocardial infarction is more serious than that which occurs with angina, and that chest pain in myocardial infarction radiates to the left arm, back, or jaw; occurs without cause, usually in the morning; is relieved only by opioids; and lasts 30 minutes or longer. Review the characteristics of the pain in myocardial infarction if you had difficulty with this question.

Level of Cognitive Ability: Analysis
Client Needs: Physiological Integrity
Integrated Process: Nursing Process/Assessment
Content Area: Physiological Adaptation

Reference
Ignatavicius D, Workman M: *Medical surgical nursing: critical thinking for collaborative care,* ed 5, Philadelphia, 2006, Saunders, p 845.

Fill-in-the-Blank

137. A physician orders 1000 mL of normal saline to infuse over 8 hours. The drop factor is 15 drops/mL. A nurse prepares to set the intravenous (IV) flow rate at how many drops per minute? (Round answer to the nearest whole number.)

Answer: _____ **drops/min**

Answer: 31

Rationale: Use the IV flow rate formula.

Formula

$$\frac{\text{Total volume} \times \text{Drop factor}}{\text{Time in minutes}} = \text{Drops/min}$$

$$\frac{1000 \text{ mL} \times 15 \text{ drops/mL}}{480 \text{ min}} = \frac{15{,}000}{480} = 31.2, \text{ or } 31 \text{ drops/min}$$

Test-Taking Strategy: Use the formula for calculating IV flow rates when answering the question. Once you have calculated the answer, verify it with a calculator. Remember to round the answer to the nearest whole number. Review IV infusion rates if you had difficulty with this question.

Level of Cognitive Ability: Application
Client Needs: Physiological Integrity
Integrated Process: Nursing Process/Implementation
Content Area: Pharmacological and Parenteral Therapies

Reference

Kee J, Marshall S: *Clinical calculations: with applications to general and specialty areas,* ed 5, Philadelphia, 2004, Saunders, p 212.

Multiple Response

138. The nurse provides dietary instructions to a client who has a folic acid deficiency. Which foods should the nurse instruct the client to consume? Select all that apply.

❏ **1** Liver
❏ **2** Eggs
❏ **3** Carrots
❏ **4** Oranges
❏ **5** Broccoli
❏ **6** Brussels sprouts

Answer: 1, 2, 5, 6

Rationale: Foods high in folic acid include liver, organ meats, eggs, cabbage, broccoli, and Brussels sprouts. Carrots are high in iron. Citrus fruits are high in vitamin B_{12} and vitamin C.

Test-Taking Strategy: Specific knowledge regarding the foods high in folic acid is needed to answer this question. Remember that foods high in folic acid include liver, organ meats, eggs, cabbage, broccoli, and Brussels sprouts. Review the foods high in folic acid if you had difficulty with this question.

Level of Cognitive Ability: Application
Client Needs: Physiological Integrity
Integrated Process: Teaching and Learning
Content Area: Basic Care and Comfort

Reference
Ignatavicius D, Workman M: *Medical-surgical nursing: critical thinking for collaborative care,* ed 5, Philadelphia, 2006, Saunders, p 894.

Multiple Response

139. The nurse monitors a client with a spinal cord injury for signs of autonomic dysreflexia. Which of the following are indications of this life-threatening syndrome? Select all that apply.

❑ **1** Piloerection
❑ **2** Tachycardia
❑ **3** Nasal stuffiness
❑ **4** Severe hypotension
❑ **5** Severe throbbing headache
❑ **6** Flushing above the level of the lesion

Answer: 1, 3, 5, 6

Rationale: Autonomic dysreflexia is characterized by a cluster of clinical manifestations that results when multiple spinal cord autonomic responses discharge simultaneously. The manifestations result from an exaggerated sympathetic response to a noxious stimulus below the level of the cord lesion. Manifestations include a sudden severe throbbing headache, severe hypertension, bradycardia, flushing above the level of the lesion (face and chest), nasal stuffiness, sweating, nausea, blurred vision, piloerection, and a feeling of apprehension.

Test-Taking Strategy: Think about the pathophysiology of autonomic dysreflexia. Recalling that it results from an exaggerated sympathetic response will assist in eliminating options 2 and 4. Review the manifestations of autonomic dysreflexia if you had difficulty with this question.

Level of Cognitive Ability: Analysis
Client Needs: Physiological Integrity
Integrated Process: Nursing Process/Assessment
Content Area: Physiological Adaptation

Reference
Ignatavicius D, Workman M: *Medical surgical nursing: critical thinking for collaborative care,* ed 5, Philadelphia, 2006, Saunders, p 988.

Multiple Response

140. The nurse is performing an assessment on a client suspected of having vitamin B_{12} deficiency. The nurse checks the client for which manifestations of this disorder? Select all that apply.

- ❏ **1** Weight loss
- ❏ **2** Slight jaundice
- ❏ **3** Facial flushing
- ❏ **4** Difficulty with gait
- ❏ **5** Smooth beefy red tongue
- ❏ **6** Paresthesia of the hands and feet

Answer: 1, 2, 4, 5, 6

Rationale: Vitamin B_{12} deficiency can occur from poor intake of foods containing vitamin B_{12} and conditions that can lead to poor absorption of vitamin B_{12}. Manifestations of this deficiency include severe pallor, slight jaundice, smooth beefy red tongue, fatigue, weight loss, paresthesia of the hands and feet, and difficulty with gait.

Test-Taking Strategy: Specific knowledge regarding the manifestations associated with vitamin B_{12} deficiency is needed to answer correctly. Also recalling the functions of vitamin B_{12} will assist in answering correctly. Remember that severe pallor, slight jaundice, smooth beefy red tongue, fatigue, weight loss, paresthesia of the hands and feet, and difficulty with gait occur in this deficiency. Review the manifestations of vitamin B_{12} deficiency if you had difficulty with this question.

Level of Cognitive Ability: Analysis
Client Needs: Physiological Integrity
Integrated Process: Nursing Process/Assessment
Content Area: Physiological Adaptation

Reference
Ignatavicius D, Workman M: *Medical surgical nursing: critical thinking for collaborative care,* ed 5, Philadelphia, 2006, Saunders, p 895.

Chart/Exhibit with a Multiple Response

141. A nurse reviews the laboratory results of an adult client and plans to report which abnormal results to the physician? Select all that apply.

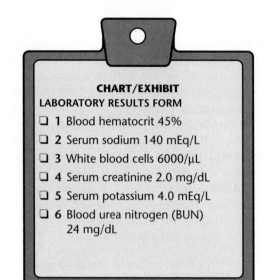

CHART/EXHIBIT
LABORATORY RESULTS FORM

❏ **1** Blood hematocrit 45%

❏ **2** Serum sodium 140 mEq/L

❏ **3** White blood cells 6000/μL

❏ **4** Serum creatinine 2.0 mg/dL

❏ **5** Serum potassium 4.0 mEq/L

❏ **6** Blood urea nitrogen (BUN) 24 mg/dL

Answer: 4, 6

Rationale: The normal serum sodium ranges from 136 to 145 mEq/L. The normal white blood cell count ranges from 4500 to 11,000/uL. The normal serum creatinine ranges from 0.8 to 1.5 mg/dL. The normal serum potassium ranges from 3.5 to 5.3 mEq/L. The normal blood hematocrit ranges from 35% to 47% (female) and 42% to 52% (male). The normal BUN ranges from 5 to 20 mg/dL.

Test-Taking Strategy: Specific knowledge regarding the normal laboratory values for the blood tests identified in the chart/exhibit is needed to answer this question. Note the strategic word *abnormal*. Therefore you are looking for the laboratory results that are not within a normal range. Review these normal values if you had difficulty with this question.

Level of Cognitive Ability: Analysis
Client Needs: Physiological Integrity
Integrated Process: Nursing Process/Assessment
Content Area: Reduction of Risk Potential

Reference
Chernecky C, Berger B: *Laboratory tests and diagnostic procedures,* ed 4, Philadelphia, 2004, Saunders, pp 428, 466, 635, 887, 1008, 1111.

Figure/Illustration with a Multiple Choice

142. The nurse understands that this type of device is used to treat which condition? (Refer to figure.)

- ❑ **1** Whiplash
- ❑ **2** Spinal stenosis
- ❑ **3** Cervical spine injury
- ❑ **4** Ruptured lumbar disk

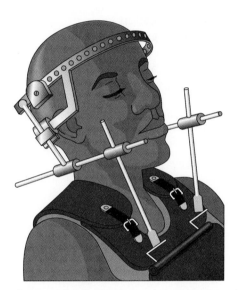

From Ignatavicius D, Workman M: *Medical surgical nursing: critical thinking for collaborative care,* ed 5, Philadelphia, 2006, Saunders.

Answer: 3

Rationale: The client with a cervical spine injury is usually placed in fixed skeletal traction to realign the vertebrae, facilitate bone healing, and prevent further injury. A whiplash injury is usually treated with a cervical collar. Spinal stenosis may be treated with exercises, massage, ultrasonic heat treatments, or transcutaneous electrical nerve stimulation. A back brace or corset is often prescribed for a client with a ruptured lumbar disk.

Test-Taking Strategy: Focus on the figure accompanying the question and note the anatomical location of the device. This will direct you to the correct option. Review the purpose and use of a halo fixation device if you had difficulty with this question.

Level of Cognitive Ability: Analysis
Client Needs: Physiological Integrity
Integrated Process: Nursing Process/Assessment
Content Area: Physiological Adaptation

References
Black J, Hawks J: *Medical-surgical nursing: clinical management for positive outcomes,* ed 7, Philadelphia, 2005, Saunders, pp 2143, 2148.
Ignatavicius D, Workman M: *Medical surgical nursing: critical thinking for collaborative care,* ed 5, Philadelphia, 2006, Saunders, pp 989-990.

Fill-in-the-Blank

143. A physician's order reads phenytoin (Dilantin) 0.1 g orally twice daily, and the medication label states 100-mg capsules. How many capsules should the nurse administer to the client to provide one dose?

Answer: _____ capsule(s)

Answer: 1

Rationale: Convert grams to milligrams and then determine the number of capsules that need to be administered. In the metric system, to convert larger to smaller, multiply by 1000 or move the decimal three places to the right. Since 0.1 g = 100 mg, the nurse administers one capsule.

Test-Taking Strategy: Focus on the data in the question and note that 0.1 g is prescribed and the medication label states 100-mg capsules. Convert grams to milligrams and then note that you will administer one capsule. Review medication calculation problems if you had difficulty with this question.

Level of Cognitive Ability: Application
Client Needs: Physiological Integrity
Integrated Process: Nursing Process/Implementation
Content Area: Pharmacological and Parenteral Therapies

Reference

Kee J, Marshall S: *Clinical calculations: with applications to general and specialty areas,* ed 5, Philadelphia, 2004, Saunders, p 22.

Multiple Response

144. A hospitalized client with heart failure suddenly develops dyspnea at rest, disorientation and confusion, and crackles in the lung bases on auscultation. Which actions should the nurse prepare to take? Select all that apply.

❑ **1** Insert a Foley catheter.
❑ **2** Monitor urinary output.
❑ **3** Administer nasal oxygen.
❑ **4** Administer a rapid-acting diuretic.
❑ **5** Place the client in a modified Trendelenburg's position.
❑ **6** Administer a 500 mL intravenous (IV) normal saline solution bolus.

Answer: 1, 2, 3, 4

Rationale: Acute pulmonary edema is a life-threatening event in which the left ventricle of the heart fails to eject sufficient blood, and pressure increases in the lungs because of the accumulated blood. Interventions are aimed at decreasing this pressure. The client is placed in a high-Fowler's position to assist in breathing. The nurse ensures that vascular access is present, but IV fluids are not administered because this will increase body fluid. Oxygen is administered, and the physician prescribes a rapid-acting diuretic to eliminate body fluid. A Foley catheter is inserted to assess urinary output after diuretic administration and to minimize exertion related to voiding.

Test-Taking Strategy: In this question it is necessary to identify three concepts: the risk for acute pulmonary edema faced by the client with heart failure, the early manifestations of acute pulmonary edema, and the treatment for acute pulmonary edema. Use the ABCs, airway, breathing, and circulation, to select option 3. Next, recall that in this condition pressure increases in the lungs because of the accumulated blood, and interventions are aimed at decreasing this pressure; this will assist in selecting options 1, 2, and 4. Review interventions for the treatment of acute pulmonary edema if you had difficulty with this question.

Level of Cognitive Ability: Application
Client Needs: Physiological Integrity
Integrated Process: Nursing Process/Implementation
Content Area: Physiological Adaptation

Reference
Ignatavicius D, Workman M: *Medical surgical nursing: critical thinking for collaborative care,* ed 5, Philadelphia, 2006, Saunders, pp 760-761.

Multiple Response

145. The nurse uses which guidelines to select a site for insertion of a peripheral venous catheter in an adult client? Select all that apply.

- ❏ 1 Choose a distal site.
- ❏ 2 Choose the client's dominant arm.
- ❏ 3 Choose an arm that is not paralyzed.
- ❏ 4 Choose a site in a vein that feels hard.
- ❏ 5 Choose a site that is away from areas of dermatitis.
- ❏ 6 Choose a site that is away from an area of joint flexion.

Answer: 1, 3, 5, 6

Rationale: Guidelines for selecting a site for insertion of a peripheral venous catheter include the following: verify the physician's order for infusion therapy; choose a site for placement in an upper extremity in an adult; choose the client's nondominant arm when possible; choose a distal site, and make all subsequent venipunctures proximal to previous sites; do not use the arm on the side of a mastectomy, lymph node dissection, or arteriovenous shunt or fistula; do not use an arm that is paralyzed; avoid choosing a site in an area of joint flexion; avoid choosing a site in a vein that is hard or cordlike (this could indicate thrombophlebitis); and avoid choosing a site close to areas of cellulitis, dermatitis, or complications from previous catheter sites.

Test-Taking Strategy: Focus on the subject, guidelines for selecting an insertion site for a peripheral venous catheter. Read each option carefully, and eliminate option 2 because of the word *dominant* and option 4 because of the word *hard.* Review these guidelines if you had difficulty with this question.

Level of Cognitive Ability: Application
Client Needs: Physiological Integrity
Integrated Process: Nursing Process/Implementation
Content Area: Pharmacological and Parenteral Therapies

Reference
Ignatavicius D, Workman M: *Medical surgical nursing: critical thinking for collaborative care,* ed 5, Philadelphia, 2006, Saunders, p 988.

Multiple Response

146. The nurse should take which immediate actions if air embolism is suspected in a client receiving intravenous therapy through a central intravenous catheter? Select all that apply.

- ❑ **1** Clamp the catheter.
- ❑ **2** Notify the physician.
- ❑ **3** Prepare to administer oxygen.
- ❑ **4** Prepare to obtain arterial blood gases.
- ❑ **5** Place the client in a high-Fowler's position.
- ❑ **6** Prepare to obtain an electrocardiogram (ECG) reading.

Answer: 1, 2, 3, 4, 6

Rationale: An air embolism occurs when air enters the central venous system during catheter insertion, tubing changes, catheter rupture, and catheter removal. Manifestations include chest pain, dyspnea, hypoxia, anxiety, tachycardia, hypotension, nausea, lightheadedness, and dizziness. A loud churning may be heard over the pericardium on auscultation. Immediate interventions include clamping the catheter; placing the client in lateral Trendelenburg's position on the left side; notifying the physician; and preparing to initiate oxygen therapy, draw arterial blood gases, and obtain an ECG reading.

Test-Taking Strategy: Focus on the subject, the interventions for an air embolism. Thinking about the pathophysiology and the cause of air embolism will assist in answering correctly. Recalling that the goal is to trap the air in the right atrium and prevent it from traveling will assist in determining that placing the client in a high-Fowler's position is incorrect. Review the manifestations of air embolism if you had difficulty with this question.

Level of Cognitive Ability: Application
Client Needs: Physiological Integrity
Integrated Process: Nursing Process/Implementation
Content Area: Pharmacological and Parenteral Therapies

Reference
Ignatavicius D, Workman M: *Medical surgical nursing: critical thinking for collaborative care,* ed 5, Philadelphia, 2006, Saunders, p 263.

Figure Illustration with a Multiple Choice

147. The nurse inspects a client's pressure ulcer and determines that the ulcer is at which stage? (Refer to figure.)

- ❏ **1** Stage I
- ❏ **2** Stage II
- ❏ **3** Stage III
- ❏ **4** Stage IV

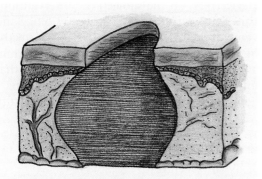

From Wilson S, Giddens J: *Health assessment for nursing practice,* ed 3, St Louis, 2005, Mosby.

Answer: 4

Rationale: In a stage IV pressure ulcer there is full-thickness skin loss with extensive destruction; tissue necrosis; or damage to muscle, bone, or supporting structures. A stage I pressure ulcer appears as a defined area of persistent redness. A stage II pressure ulcer is a partial-thickness skin loss involving the epidermis, dermis, or both; is superficial; and appears as an abrasion, blister, or shallow crater. A stage III pressure ulcer involves damage to or necrosis of subcutaneous tissue that may extend down to, but not through, underlying fascia and appears as a deep crater.

Test-Taking Strategy: Focus on the figure provided with this question. Note the full-thickness skin loss with destruction to underlying structures. This will direct you to the correct option. Review the stages of pressure ulcers if you had difficulty with this question.

Level of Cognitive Ability: Analysis
Client Needs: Physiological Integrity
Integrated Process: Nursing Process/Assessment
Content Area: Physiological Adaptation

Reference
Wilson S, Giddens J: *Health assessment for nursing practice,* ed 3, St Louis, 2005, Mosby, p 187.

Fill-in-the-Blank

148. A physician orders 1 unit of packed red blood cells to infuse over 4 hours. The unit of blood contains 250 mL. The drop factor is 15 drops/mL. A nurse prepares to set the intravenous (IV) flow rate at how many drops per minute? (Round answer to the nearest whole number.)

Answer: _____ **drops/min**

Answer: 16

Rationale: Use the IV flow rate formula.

Formula

$$\frac{\text{Total volume} \times \text{Drop factor}}{\text{Time in minutes}} = \text{Drops/min}$$

$$\frac{250 \text{ mL} \times 15 \text{ drops/mL}}{240 \text{ min}} = \frac{3750}{240} = 15.6, \text{ or } 16 \text{ drops/min}$$

Test-Taking Strategy: Use the formula for calculating IV flow rates when answering the question. Once you have calculated the answer, verify it with a calculator. Remember to round the answer to the nearest whole number. Review IV infusion rates if you had difficulty with this question.

Level of Cognitive Ability: Application
Client Needs: Physiological Integrity
Integrated Process: Nursing Process/Implementation
Content Area: Pharmacological and Parenteral Therapies

Reference
Kee J, Marshall S: *Clinical calculations: with applications to general and specialty areas,* ed 5, Philadelphia, 2004, Saunders, p 212.

Multiple Response

149. The nurse is preparing to administer a medication by the Z-track method and takes which actions to prepare and administer the medication? Select all that apply.

- ❑ 1 Use a 25-gauge, 1-inch long needle.
- ❑ 2 Massage the injection site after administration.
- ❑ 3 Select the dorsogluteal site (upper outer quadrant) for the injection.
- ❑ 4 Add 0.25 mL of air to the syringe after drawing up the medication.
- ❑ 5 Aspirate to determine needle placement before administering the medication.
- ❑ 6 Place a new needle on the syringe after the medication is drawn into the syringe.

Answer: 3, 4, 5, 6

Rationale: The Z-track method of injection is used for medications that need to be deposited deep into the muscle or for medications that can stain the tissues and skin. An example of a medication that is administered by this method is an iron solution. The procedure for administering medication by this method is as follows: (1) draw the medication into the syringe using aseptic technique; (2) add 0.25 mL air to the syringe (air lock); (3) discard the needle used to draw up the medication; (4) place a new needle (22-gauge, 2 to 3 inches long) on the syringe; (5) select the dorsogluteal site only (upper outer quadrant); (6) pull the skin and subcutaneous tissue sideways away from the muscle; (7) clean the site while holding the skin and subcutaneous tissue off to the side; (8) insert the needle deeply into the muscle tissue; (9) aspirate to determine needle placement (withdraw the needle and begin the procedure again from the first step if blood is aspirated); (10) inject the medication, followed by injection of the air bubble; and (11) release the skin and subcutaneous tissue. The injection site is not massaged.

Test-Taking Strategy: Focus on the subject, the Z-track method of medication administration. Remember that the Z-track method is used for injecting medications that need to be deposited deep into the muscle or for medications that can stain the tissues and skin. With this in mind, visualize each of the actions in the options to direct you to the correct answers. Review the Z-track method of injection if you had difficulty with this question.

Level of Cognitive Ability: Application
Client Needs: Physiological Integrity
Integrated Process: Nursing Process/Implementation
Content Area: Pharmacological and Parenteral Therapies

Reference
Ignatavicius D, Workman M: *Medical surgical nursing: critical thinking for collaborative care,* ed 5, Philadelphia, 2006, Saunders, p 894.

Multiple Response

150. The nurse develops a care plan for a client with thrombocytopenia. The nurse includes which interventions in the plan of care? Select all that apply.

❏ **1** Apply heat to all areas of trauma.
❏ **2** Avoid giving the client hard food.
❏ **3** Take axillary or tympanic temperatures.
❏ **4** Monitor the client for signs of bleeding.
❏ **5** Provide the client with an electric razor.
❏ **6** Instruct the client to avoid flossing the teeth.

Answer: 2, 3, 4, 5, 6

Rationale: Thrombocytopenia is a condition in which the number of circulating platelets is reduced, placing the client at risk for bleeding. The nurse must implement bleeding precautions, including monitoring the client for signs of bleeding; handling the client gently; avoiding injections and venipunctures as much as possible and using the smallest gauge needle possible if injections and venipunctures are necessary; applying firm pressure to a needlestick site for 5 to 10 minutes or until the site no longer oozes blood; applying ice to all areas of trauma; avoiding rectal temperatures, enemas, and suppositories; using an electric razor; avoiding mouth trauma by using a soft-bristled toothbrush and avoiding flossing or chewing on hard food; avoiding nose blowing; and avoiding contact sports.

Test-Taking Strategy: Recall that thrombocytopenia places the client at risk for bleeding. Read each option, noting whether it presents a risk for bleeding. Using principles about the effects of heat and cold will assist in eliminating option 1. Review interventions for a client at risk for bleeding if you had difficulty with this question.

Level of Cognitive Ability: Application
Client Needs: Physiological Integrity
Integrated Process: Nursing Process/Planning
Content Area: Physiological Adaptation

Reference
Ignatavicius D, Workman M: *Medical surgical nursing: critical thinking for collaborative care,* ed 5, Philadelphia, 2006, Saunders, p 906.

Prioritizing (Ordered Response)

151. Identify the steps in order of priority for inserting a nasogastric tube. (Number 1 is the first step and number 6 is the last step.)

____ Verify tube placement.
____ Anchor the tube to the nose.
____ Position the client in high-Fowler's position.
____ Document the tube length in the client's record.
____ Measure the distance to insert the tube and mark the length of the tube; lubricate the end of the tube with water-soluble lubricating jelly.
____ Insert the tube through the naris and instruct the client to take a sip of water and swallow, continuing to advance the tube until the tape mark is reached.

Answer: 4, 5, 1, 6, 2, 3

Rationale: To insert a nasogastric tube, the nurse first performs hand hygiene and explains the procedure to the client. The nurse applies gloves and positions the client in high-Fowler's position, then places a bath towel over the client's chest. The nurse next measures the distance to insert the tube (the distance from the tip of the nose to the earlobe to the xiphoid process), marks the length of the tube, and lubricates the end of the tube with water-soluble lubricating jelly. The nurse inserts the tube through the naris and, with the tube just above the oropharynx, instructs the client to flex the head forward and take a sip of water and swallow. The nurse continues to advance the tube until the tape mark is reached. The nurse then verifies tube placement and anchors the tube to the nose. Once the procedure is complete, the nurse documents the tube length and other appropriate data in the client's record.

Test-Taking Strategy: Visualize this procedure to assist in determining the correct order of action. Remember that the nurse positions the client before measuring the tube and inserting the tube and documents once the procedure is complete. Review this procedure if you had difficulty with this question.

Level of Cognitive Ability: Application
Client Needs: Physiological Integrity
Integrated Process: Nursing Process/Implementation
Content Area: Physiological Adaptation

Reference
Black J, Hawks J: *Medical-surgical nursing: clinical management for positive outcomes,* ed 7, Philadelphia, 2005, Saunders, pp 1404-1405.

Figure/Illustration with a Multiple Choice

152. While providing care to a client, the nurse notes that a client exhibits this posture (see figure). The nurse documents that the client is exhibiting which of the following?

❑ **1** Flaccidity
❑ **2** Decorticate posturing
❑ **3** Decerebrate posturing
❑ **4** Rigidity in the upper extremities

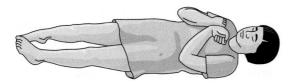

From Ignatavicius D, Workman M: *Medical surgical nursing: critical thinking for collaborative care,* ed 5, Philadelphia, 2006, Saunders.

Answer: 2

Rationale: Decortication is abnormal posturing seen in the client with lesions that interrupt the corticospinal pathways. In this posturing the client's arms, wrists, and fingers are flexed with internal rotation and plantar flexion of the legs. Decerebration is abnormal posturing and rigidity characterized by extension of the arms and legs, pronation of the arms, plantar flexion, and opisthotonos. Decerebration is usually associated with dysfunction in the brainstem area. Flaccidity indicates weak, soft, and flabby muscles that lack normal muscle tone. Rigidity indicates hardness, stiffness, or inflexibility. Decerebrate posturing is associated with rigidity.

Test-Taking Strategy: Focus on the figure and use knowledge regarding the characteristics of posturing to answer the question. First eliminate options 3 and 4 because they are comparative or alike in that decerebrate posturing is associated with rigidity. Next, recalling that flaccidity indicates weak, soft, and flabby muscles that lack normal muscle tone will assist in eliminating option 1. Review the characteristics of posturing if you had difficulty with this question.

Level of Cognitive Ability: Analysis
Client Needs: Physiological Integrity
Integrated Process: Nursing Process/Assessment
Content Area: Physiological Adaptation

Reference
Ignatavicius D, Workman M: *Medical surgical nursing: critical thinking for collaborative care,* ed 5, Philadelphia, 2006, Saunders, p 939.

Multiple Response

153. A client admitted to the hospital is suspected of having Guillain-Barré syndrome. The nurse reviews the client's medical record, expecting to note documentation of which manifestations of this disorder? Select all that apply.

❑ **1** Dysphagia
❑ **2** Paresthesia
❑ **3** Facial weakness
❑ **4** Difficulty speaking
❑ **5** Hyperactive deep tendon reflexes
❑ **6** Descending symmetrical muscle weakness

Answer: 1, 2, 3, 4

Rationale: Guillain-Barré syndrome is an acute autoimmune disorder characterized by varying degrees of motor weakness and paralysis. Motor manifestations include ascending symmetrical muscle weakness that leads to flaccid paralysis without muscle atrophy, decreased or absent deep tendon reflexes, respiratory compromise and respiratory failure, and loss of bladder and bowel control. Sensory manifestations include pain (cramping) and paresthesia. Cranial nerve manifestations include facial weakness, dysphagia, diplopia, and difficulty speaking. Autonomic manifestations include labile blood pressure, dysrhythmias, and tachycardia.

Test-Taking Strategy: Focus on the client's diagnosis and recall that Guillain-Barré syndrome is an acute autoimmune disorder characterized by varying degrees of motor weakness and paralysis. This will assist in determining that options 1, 2, 3, and 4 are correct. To remember the progression of paralysis that occurs in this disorder, think about *G to B* (Guillain-Barré), from the *G*round to the *B*rain. Review the manifestations of this disorder if you had difficulty with this question.

Level of Cognitive Ability: Analysis
Client Needs: Physiological Integrity
Integrated Process: Nursing Process/Assessment
Content Area: Physiological Adaptation

Reference
Ignatavicius D, Workman M: *Medical surgical nursing: critical thinking for collaborative care,* ed 5, Philadelphia, 2006, Saunders, p 1008.

Multiple Response

154. The nurse provides home care instructions for a client with peripheral neuropathy of the lower extremities. The nurse includes which instructions in the plan? Select all that apply.

- ❑ **1** Wear support or elastic stockings.
- ❑ **2** Wear well-fitted shoes and walk barefoot only when at home.
- ❑ **3** Use a heating pad set at low setting on the feet if they feel cold.
- ❑ **4** Wear dark-colored stockings or socks and change them daily.
- ❑ **5** Apply lanolin or lubricating lotion to the legs and feet once or twice daily.
- ❑ **6** Wash the feet and legs with mild soap and water and rinse and dry them well.

Answer: 1, 5, 6

Rationale: Peripheral neuropathy is any functional or organic disorder of the peripheral nervous system. Clinical manifestations can include muscle weakness, stabbing pain, paresthesia or loss of sensation, impaired reflexes, and autonomic manifestations. Home care instructions include washing the feet and legs with mild soap and water and rinsing and drying them well, applying lanolin or lubricating lotion to the legs and feet once or twice daily, inspecting the legs and feet daily and reporting any skin changes or open areas to the physician, wearing white or colorfast stockings or socks and changing them daily, checking the temperature of the bath water with a thermometer before putting the feet into the water, avoiding the use of heat (hot foot soaks, heating pad, hot water bottle) on the feet because of the risk of burning, avoiding the use of sharp devices to cut nails, wearing support or elastic stockings for dependent edema, and wearing well-fitted shoes and avoiding going barefoot.

Test-Taking Strategy: Focus on the client's diagnosis and recall that the client with peripheral neuropathy experiences paresthesia or loss of sensation. This will assist in eliminating option 3. Next eliminate option 2 because of the close-ended word *only*. Finally eliminate option 4 because the client needs to wear white or colorfast stockings or socks. Review home care instructions for a client with peripheral neuropathy if you had difficulty with this question.

Level of Cognitive Ability: Application
Client Needs: Physiological Integrity
Integrated Process: Teaching and Learning
Content Area: Reduction of Risk Potential

Reference
Ignatavicius D, Workman M: *Medical surgical nursing: critical thinking for collaborative care,* ed 5, Philadelphia, 2006, Saunders, p 1020.

Multiple Response

155. A client comes into the health care clinic stating that she thinks she has restless leg syndrome. The nurse assesses the client knowing that which of the following are characteristics of this disorder? Select all that apply.

    ❑ 1 A heavy feeling in the legs
    ❑ 2 Burning sensations in the limbs
    ❑ 3 Symptom relief when lying down
    ❑ 4 Decreased ability to move the legs
    ❑ 5 Symptoms that are worse in the morning
    ❑ 6 Feeling the need to move the limbs repeatedly

Answer: 2, 6

Rationale: Restless leg syndrome is characterized by leg paresthesia associated with an irresistible urge to move. The client complains of intense burning or "crawling-type" sensations in the limbs and subsequently feels the need to move the limbs repeatedly. The symptoms are worse in the evening and night when the client is still. The client feels the need to move to relieve the symptoms.

Test-Taking Strategy: Focus on the name of the disorder, *restless leg syndrome.* This will assist in eliminating options 1, 3, 4. Next recall that the symptoms of this disorder are worse in the evening and night when the client is still. Review the characteristics of restless leg syndrome if you had difficulty with this question.

Level of Cognitive Ability: Analysis
Client Needs: Physiological Integrity
Integrated Process: Nursing Process/Assessment
Content Area: Physiological Adaptation

Reference
Ignatavicius D, Workman M: *Medical surgical nursing: critical thinking for collaborative care,* ed 5, Philadelphia, 2006, Saunders, p 1022.

Multiple Response

156. A client diagnosed with Bell's palsy asks the nurse about the disorder. The nurse provides the client with which information? Select all that apply.

❏ 1 It is an acute paralysis of cranial nerve VII.
❏ 2 The client should eat and drink using the unaffected side of the face.
❏ 3 It may occur as a result of an inflammatory process.
❏ 4 The application of warm moist heat may alleviate discomfort.
❏ 5 Facial exercises and massage need to be avoided to prevent damage to facial tissues.
❏ 6 It always occurs bilaterally, and in about 1 week both sides of the face will be affected.

Answer: 1, 2, 3, 4

Rationale: Bell's palsy is an acute paralysis of cranial nerve VII and may occur as a result of an inflammatory process. Pain behind the ear or on the face may precede paralysis by a few hours or days. The disorder is characterized by a drawing sensation and paralysis of all facial muscles on the affected side. The client cannot close the eye, wrinkle the forehead, smile, whistle, or grimace. The face appears masklike and sags. The client is encouraged to eat and drink using the unaffected side of the face. Simple techniques of massage, the application of warm moist heat to alleviate discomfort, and facial exercises may be helpful to maintain muscle tone.

Test-Taking Strategy: Read each option carefully. Recalling that Bell's palsy occurs on one side of the face will assist in eliminating option 6. Also note the close-ended word *always* in this option. Next think about the effects of the disorder and recall that one goal of therapy is to preserve muscle tone; this will assist in eliminating option 5. Review the characteristics of Bell's palsy if you had difficulty with this question.

Level of Cognitive Ability: Application
Client Needs: Physiological Integrity
Integrated Process: Nursing Process/Implementation
Content Area: Physiological Adaptation

Reference
Ignatavicius D, Workman M: *Medical surgical nursing: critical thinking for collaborative care,* ed 5, Philadelphia, 2006, Saunders, p 1024.

Multiple Response

157. The nurse assesses a client for risk factors associated with a brain attack (stroke). Which of the following are risk factors? Select all that apply.

- ❑ **1** Smoking
- ❑ **2** Underweight
- ❑ **3** Hypertension
- ❑ **4** Active lifestyle
- ❑ **5** Diabetes mellitus
- ❑ **6** Oral contraceptive use

Answer: 1, 3, 5, 6

Rationale: A stroke is caused by a disruption in the normal blood supply to the brain. Some of the risk factors for stroke are hypertension; diabetes mellitus; smoking; obesity; sedentary lifestyle; oral contraceptive use; elevated cholesterol levels; heavy alcohol use; hereditary or familial tendency; atrial fibrillation, myocardial infarction, valvular heart disease, or other heart disease; illicit drug use; and hypercoagulable conditions.

Test-Taking Strategy: Recall that a stroke is caused by a disruption in the normal blood supply to the brain. Think about the causes of this disruption and the effects of each of the options on this disruption. This will assist in answering the question. Review the risk factors associated with stroke if you had difficulty with this question.

Level of Cognitive Ability: Analysis
Client Needs: Physiological Integrity
Integrated Process: Nursing Process/Assessment
Content Area: Physiological Adaptation

Reference
Ignatavicius D, Workman M: *Medical surgical nursing: critical thinking for collaborative care,* ed 5, Philadelphia, 2006, Saunders, p 1031.

Multiple Response

158. The nurse is told in report that an assigned client suffered a right cerebral hemisphere brain attack (stroke). The nurse expects to note which manifestations on assessment of the client? Select all that apply.

- ❏ 1 Impulsiveness
- ❏ 2 Problems reading
- ❏ 3 Difficulty writing
- ❏ 4 Neglect of the left visual field
- ❏ 5 Inability to comprehend language
- ❏ 6 Disorientation to time, place, and person

Answer: 1, 4, 6

Rationale: A right cerebral hemisphere stroke affects visual and spatial awareness and proprioception. The client is often unaware of any deficits and may be disoriented to time, place, and person. Manifestations include visual spatial deficits, neglect of the left visual field, and loss of depth perception; disorientation to time, place, and person and inability to recognize faces; loss of the ability to hear tonal variations; and an impaired sense of humor. Behavioral manifestations include impulsiveness, lack of awareness of the neurological deficit, confabulation, euphoria, constant smiling, denial of illness, poor judgment, and overestimation of abilities (which places the client at risk for injury). The left cerebral hemisphere is the center for language, mathematical skills, and analytic thinking. A left hemispheric stroke results in aphasia (inability to use or comprehend language), alexia (reading problems), and agraphia (difficulty with writing). The client with a left hemispheric stroke tends to be slow and cautious.

Test-Taking Strategy: Focus on the subject, a right cerebral hemisphere stroke. Recalling the functions of the right cerebral hemisphere will direct you to the correct options. Review the characteristics of both right and left cerebral hemisphere strokes if you had difficulty with this question.

Level of Cognitive Ability: Analysis
Client Needs: Physiological Integrity
Integrated Process: Nursing Process/Assessment
Content Area: Physiological Adaptation

Reference
Ignatavicius D, Workman M: *Medical surgical nursing: critical thinking for collaborative care,* ed 5, Philadelphia, 2006, Saunders, p 1034.

Multiple Response

159. The nurse monitors a client who experienced a head injury. Which of the following manifestations indicates to the nurse an increase in intracranial pressure (ICP)? Select all that apply.

❑ **1** Hypotension
❑ **2** Restlessness
❑ **3** Tachycardia
❑ **4** Pupillary changes
❑ **5** Abnormal posturing
❑ **6** Widened pulse pressure

Answer: 2, 4, 5, 6

Rationale: ICP is the pressure that occurs within the cranium. The first sign of increased ICP is a decline in the level of consciousness. Other manifestations of increased ICP include behavior changes such as restless, irritability, and confusion; headache; nausea and vomiting; changes in speech pattern, aphasia, or slurred speech; pupillary changes; cranial nerve dysfunction; ataxia; seizures; Cushing's triad (severe hypertension, widened pulse pressure, and bradycardia); and abnormal posturing.

Test-Taking Strategy: Recall that increased ICP indicates increased pressure within the cranium. Recalling that this occurrence will affect neurological status will assist in determining that options 2, 4, and 5 are correct. From the remaining options, recall Cushing's triad (severe hypertension, widened pulse pressure, and bradycardia) to answer correctly. Review the manifestations of increased ICP if you had difficulty with this question.

Level of Cognitive Ability: Analysis
Client Needs: Physiological Integrity
Integrated Process: Nursing Process/Assessment
Content Area: Physiological Adaptation

Reference

Ignatavicius D, Workman M: *Medical surgical nursing: critical thinking for collaborative care,* ed 5, Philadelphia, 2006, Saunders, p 1037.

Multiple Response

160. The nurse notes documentation that a client who experienced a brain attack (stroke) has receptive aphasia. The nurse expects to note which characteristics of this type of aphasia in the client? Select all that apply.

❏ 1 Has difficulty writing
❏ 2 Has meaningless speech
❏ 3 Has difficulty forming words
❏ 4 Makes up words when speaking
❏ 5 Has difficulty understanding spoken words
❏ 6 Has difficulty understanding written words

Answer: 2, 4, 5, 6

Rationale: Receptive (Wernicke's or sensory) aphasia is due to injury involving Wernicke's area in the temporoparietal area. The client is unable to understand spoken and, often, written words. The client's language is often meaningless and commonly contains neologisms (made-up words). Expressive (Broca's or motor) aphasia is the result of damage to Broca's area of the frontal lobe. It is a motor speech problem in which the client generally understands what is said but is unable to communicate verbally. The client has difficulty writing, is aware of the deficit, and may become frustrated and angry. Global or mixed aphasia occurs when the client exhibits dysfunction in both expression and reception.

Test-Taking Strategy: Focus on the subject, receptive aphasia. Recalling that receptive aphasia is a sensory aphasia and is due to injury involving Wernicke's area in the temporoparietal area will assist in determining that options 2, 4, 5, and 6 are correct. Review the types of aphasia and their characteristics if you had difficulty with this question.

Level of Cognitive Ability: Analysis
Client Needs: Physiological Integrity
Integrated Process: Nursing Process/Assessment
Content Area: Physiological Adaptation

Reference
Ignatavicius D, Workman M: *Medical surgical nursing: critical thinking for collaborative care,* ed 5, Philadelphia, 2006, Saunders, p 1043.

Multiple Response

161. The nurse is performing an assessment on an older client. Which of the following are age-related changes in the eye? Select all that apply.

- ❏ **1** Clear sclera
- ❏ **2** Blurred vision
- ❏ **3** Protruding cornea
- ❏ **4** Increased tear production
- ❏ **5** Diminished pupillary adaptation to darkness
- ❏ **6** Increased ability to discriminate among colors

Answer: 2, 5

Rationale: Age-related changes in the eye include a sunken appearance; yellowing sclera; flattening of the cornea, which causes blurred vision; reduced ocular muscle strength; poor pupillary adaptation to darkness; diminished ability to discriminate among colors; and diminished tear production.

Test-Taking Strategy: Focus on the subject, age-related changes in the eye. Eliminate options 4 and 6 because of the word *increased*. From the remaining options recall that age-related changes include yellowing sclera, flattening of the cornea, blurred vision, and poor pupillary adaptation to darkness. Review these age-related changes if you had difficulty with this question.

Level of Cognitive Ability: Analysis
Client Needs: Physiological Integrity
Integrated Process: Nursing Process/Assessment
Content Area: Physiological Adaptation

Reference
Ignatavicius D, Workman M: *Medical surgical nursing: critical thinking for collaborative care,* ed 5, Philadelphia, 2006, Saunders, p 1075

Multiple Response

162. A client is diagnosed with cataracts. The nurse reviews the client's medical record and expects to note documentation of which manifestations of this disorder? Select all that apply.

- ❑ **1** Diplopia
- ❑ **2** Blurred vision
- ❑ **3** Absent red reflex
- ❑ **4** Reduced visual acuity
- ❑ **5** Presence of a white pupil
- ❑ **6** Increased color perception

Answer: 1, 2, 3, 4, 5

Rationale: A cataract is an opacity of the lens of the eye that distorts the image projected onto the retina. Manifestations include blurred vision, decreased color perception, diplopia, reduced visual acuity (which can progress to blindness), absent red reflex, and the presence of a white pupil.

Test-Taking Strategy: Recall that a cataract is an opacity of the lens of the eye that distorts the image projected onto the retina. This will assist in selecting options 1, 2, and 4. From the remaining options focus on the description of a cataract and remember that absent red reflex and the presence of a white pupil are clinical manifestations. Review the manifestations of a cataract if you had difficulty with this question.

Level of Cognitive Ability: Analysis
Client Needs: Physiological Integrity
Integrated Process: Nursing Process/Assessment
Content Area: Physiological Adaptation

Reference
Ignatavicius D, Workman M: *Medical surgical nursing: critical thinking for collaborative care,* ed 5, Philadelphia, 2006, Saunders, p 1093.

Multiple Response

163. The nurse provides information to a client who had cataract surgery about the activities that increase intraocular pressure (IOP). Which of the following activities will increase IOP? Select all that apply.

❑ **1** Vomiting
❑ **2** Blowing the nose
❑ **3** Bending at the knees
❑ **4** Sneezing or coughing
❑ **5** Keeping the head elevated
❑ **6** Straining to have a bowel movement

Answer: 1, 2, 4, 6

Rationale: Increased IOP is a major complication following cataract surgery, and the nurse provides the client information about the activities to avoid to prevent this increase. Activities that increase IOP include bending from the waist, sneezing or coughing, blowing the nose, straining to have a bowel movement, vomiting, having sexual intercourse, keeping the head in a dependent position, and wearing shirts with tight collars.

Test-Taking Strategy: Focus on the subject, activities that increase IOP. Read each option and think about how the activity may or may not increase pressure. This will assist in eliminating options 3 and 5. Review postoperative instructions following cataract surgery and the activities that increase IOP if you had difficulty with this question.

Level of Cognitive Ability: Application
Client Needs: Physiological Integrity
Integrated Process: Teaching and Learning
Content Area: Physiological Adaptation

Reference
Ignatavicius D, Workman M: *Medical surgical nursing: critical thinking for collaborative care,* ed 5, Philadelphia, 2006, Saunders, p 1095.

Multiple Response

164. A client is diagnosed with glaucoma. The nurse reviews the client's medical record, expecting to note which of the following? Select all that apply.

❑ **1** Halos around lights
❑ **2** Headache or eye pain
❑ **3** Decreased visual acuity
❑ **4** Loss of peripheral vision
❑ **5** Increased accommodation
❑ **6** Tonometry reading of 24 mm Hg

Answer: 1, 2, 3, 4, 6

Rationale: Glaucoma is a group of ocular diseases resulting in increased intraocular pressure (IOP). IOP is the fluid (aqueous humor) pressure within the eye. A normal IOP is 10 to 21 mm Hg and is maintained when there is a balance between production and outflow of aqueous humor. Early manifestations of glaucoma include increased IOP and diminished accommodation. Late manifestations include diminished visual fields (loss of peripheral vision), decreased visual acuity not correctable with glasses, halos around lights, headache or eye pain, and a pale optic disc.

Test-Taking Strategy: Focus on the diagnosis and recall that glaucoma results in increased IOP. Focusing on this description, eliminate option 5 because of the word *increased*. Review the manifestations of glaucoma if you had difficulty with this question.

Level of Cognitive Ability: Analysis
Client Needs: Physiological Integrity
Integrated Process: Nursing Process/Assessment
Content Area: Physiological Adaptation

Reference
Ignatavicius D, Workman M: *Medical surgical nursing: critical thinking for collaborative care,* ed 5, Philadelphia, 2006, Saunders, p 1097.

Multiple Response

165. An older client is diagnosed with macular degeneration and asks the nurse to describe this condition. The nurse includes which information in the response to the client? Select all that apply.

- ❑ **1** It can be an age-related problem.
- ❑ **2** Mild blurring and distortion occur.
- ❑ **3** It is caused by gradual blockage of retinal capillaries.
- ❑ **4** It is a deterioration of the area that controls peripheral vision.
- ❑ **5** Treatment aims to help the client maximize remaining vision.
- ❑ **6** There are two types, atropic (age related, or dry) or exudative (wet).

Answer: 1, 2, 3, 5, 6

Rationale: Macular degeneration is a deterioration of the macula, the area of central vision. It can be atropic (age related, or dry) or exudative (wet). Age-related degeneration is caused by gradual blockage of retinal capillaries, allowing retinal cells in the macula to become ischemic and necrotic. Rod and cone photoreceptors die. Central vision declines, and the client complains of mild blurring and distortion. Treatment of age-related macular degeneration aims to help the client maximize remaining vision. Management of clients with exudative macular degeneration is geared toward slowing the process and identifying further changes in visual perception.

Test-Taking Strategy: Read each option carefully. Recalling that macular degeneration is a deterioration of the macula, the area of central vision, will assist in eliminating the only incorrect option, option 4. Review the characteristics of macular degeneration if you had difficulty with this question.

Level of Cognitive Ability: Application
Client Needs: Physiological Integrity
Integrated Process: Teaching and Learning
Content Area: Physiological Adaptation

Reference

Ignatavicius D, Workman M: *Medical surgical nursing: critical thinking for collaborative care,* ed 5, Philadelphia, 2006, Saunders, p 1102.

Multiple Response

166. A client sustained a penetrating eye injury from a piece of glass when a mirror with a metal backing in the client's bathroom fell and broke. On visual assessment of the injured eye, the nurse can see a piece of glass protruding from the eye. The nurse prepares the client for which interventions? Select all that apply.

❏ **1** X-rays studies of the orbit
❏ **2** Assessment of visual acuity
❏ **3** Administration of a tetanus booster
❏ **4** Immediate removal of the glass with forceps
❏ **5** Computed tomography (CT) scans of the orbit
❏ **6** Magnetic resonance imaging (MRI) of the eye orbit

Answer: 1, 2, 3, 5

Rationale: If the client sustains a penetrating eye injury, the nurse does not remove the object. It is removed only by the ophthalmologist, since the object may be holding eye structures in place. X-ray and CT scans of the orbit are usually performed to ensure that the orbit is intact and to look for fractures that might entrap orbital muscles. MRI is contraindicated because the procedure may move any metal-containing object and cause more injury. The nurse would assess and document visual acuity and administer a tetanus booster if needed.

Test-Taking Strategy: Focus on the injury and note the strategic words *protruding from the eye* and *metal backing*. These words will assist in eliminating options 4 and 6. Review care to the client with a penetrating eye injury if you had difficulty with this question.

Level of Cognitive Ability: Application
Client Needs: Physiological Integrity
Integrated Process: Nursing Process/Implementation
Content Area: Physiological Adaptation

Reference
Ignatavicius D, Workman M: *Medical surgical nursing: critical thinking for collaborative care,* ed 5, Philadelphia, 2006, Saunders, p 1106.

Multiple Response

167. The nurse provides postoperative instructions to a client who had a myringotomy and tells the client which of the following? Select all that apply.

- ❏ **1** Use a straw for drinking.
- ❏ **2** Avoid bending-over activities.
- ❏ **3** Avoid rapid movements of the head.
- ❏ **4** Avoid straining when having a bowel movement.
- ❏ **5** Blow the nose gently, one side at a time, with the mouth open.
- ❏ **6** Excessive ear drainage is expected and is nothing to be concerned about.

Answer: 2, 3, 4, 5

Rationale: A myringotomy is the surgical opening of the pars tensa of the eardrum to drain middle ear fluids. After ear surgery the client is instructed to avoid straining when having a bowel movement and to avoid drinking through a straw, air travel, and excessive coughing for 2 to 3 weeks. Additional instructions include staying away from individuals with colds; blowing the nose gently, one side at a time, with the mouth open; avoiding wetting the head and showering for 1 week; keeping the ear dry for 6 weeks by placing a ball of cotton coated with petroleum jelly in the ear (this should be changed daily); avoiding rapid movements of the head, bouncing, and bending over for 3 weeks; and reporting excessive drainage to the physician immediately.

Test-Taking Strategy: Focus on the subject, client instructions following ear surgery. Recall that any activity that increases pressure in the operative site needs to be avoided. This will assist in eliminating option 1. Noting the word *excessive* in option 6 will assist in eliminating this option. Review postoperative instructions following ear surgery if you had difficulty with this question.

Level of Cognitive Ability: Application
Client Needs: Physiological Integrity
Integrated Process: Teaching and Learning
Content Area: Reduction of Risk Potential

Reference

Ignatavicius D, Workman M: *Medical surgical nursing: critical thinking for collaborative care,* ed 5, Philadelphia, 2006, Saunders, p 1130.

Multiple Response

168. A client is diagnosed with Meniere's disease and asks the nurse to describe the disorder. The nurse provides the client with which information? Select all that apply.

❑ **1** Ringing in the ears occurs.
❑ **2** It is characterized by vertigo.
❑ **3** Bilateral sensorineural hearing loss occurs.
❑ **4** Permanent hearing loss develops as the attacks increase.
❑ **5** Cigarette smoking is stopped because of the blood vessel–constricting effect.
❑ **6** Salt and fluid restrictions that reduce the amount of fluid in the ear may be helpful.

Answer: 1, 2, 4, 5, 6

Rationale: Meniere's disease occurs as a result of either over-production or decreased reabsorption of endolymphatic fluid. The characteristic features include tinnitus, one-sided sensori-neural hearing loss, and vertigo, occurring in attacks that can last for several days. In the early stages, periods of remission are marked by normal or nearly normal hearing, but permanent hearing loss develops as the attacks increase. Dietary and lifestyle changes such as salt and fluid restrictions that reduce the amount of endolymphatic fluid may be helpful. Cigarette smoking is stopped because of the blood vessel–constricting effect. Medications are prescribed to control the vertigo and vomiting and restore normal balance. Mild diuretics may also be prescribed. Surgical treatment of the disease is a last resort because surgery further affects hearing.

Test-Taking Strategy: Read each option carefully and think about the pathophysiology of this disorder. Recall that the characteristic features include tinnitus, one-sided sensorineural hearing loss, and vertigo. This will assist in eliminating option 3. Also remember that permanent hearing loss develops as the attacks increase and that treatment includes stopping cigarette smoking and restricting salt and fluids. Review the characteristics of Meniere's disease if you had difficulty with this question.

Level of Cognitive Ability: Application
Client Needs: Physiological Integrity
Integrated Process: Teaching and Learning
Content Area: Physiological Adaptation

Reference
Ignatavicius D, Workman M: *Medical surgical nursing: critical thinking for collaborative care,* ed 5, Philadelphia, 2006, Saunders, p 1133.

Multiple Response

169. The nurse monitors a client with a pelvic fracture sustained in an automobile crash for signs of fat embolism syndrome. Which of the following manifestations are indicative of this complication? Select all that apply.

- ❑ **1** Dyspnea
- ❑ **2** Chest pain
- ❑ **3** Bradypnea
- ❑ **4** Bradycardia
- ❑ **5** Lung crackles
- ❑ **6** Altered mental status

Answer: 1, 2, 5, 6

Rationale: Fat embolism syndrome is a serious complication resulting from a fracture in which fat globules are released from the normal bone marrow into the bloodstream. Manifestations include altered mental status (earliest sign caused by a low arterial oxygen level); increased respirations, pulse, and temperature; chest pain, dyspnea, and lung crackles; decreased Sao_2; and petechiae.

Test-Taking Strategy: Think about the pathophysiology of an embolism. This will assist in eliminating options 3 and 4. Remember that increased respirations, pulse, and temperature occur in fat embolism syndrome. Review the manifestations of fat embolism syndrome if you had difficulty with this question.

Level of Cognitive Ability: Analysis
Client Needs: Physiological Integrity
Integrated Process: Nursing Process/Assessment
Content Area: Physiological Adaptation

Reference

Ignatavicius D, Workman M: *Medical surgical nursing: critical thinking for collaborative care,* ed 5, Philadelphia, 2006, Saunders, p 1193.

Multiple Response

170. The nurse develops a postprocedure care plan for a client scheduled for colonoscopy. The nurse includes which of the following in the immediate postprocedure care plan? Select all that apply.

- ❏ 1 Keep the side rails up.
- ❏ 2 Maintain an NPO status.
- ❏ 3 Assess for rectal bleeding and clots.
- ❏ 4 Take vital signs every 15 to 30 minutes.
- ❏ 5 Monitor for manifestations of bowel perforation and hypovolemic shock.
- ❏ 6 Inform the client that fullness and mild abdominal cramping need to be reported to the physician immediately.

Answer: 1, 2, 3, 4, 5

Rationale: A colonoscopy is an endoscopic examination of the entire large bowel. In this procedure the physician may obtain tissue biopsy specimens or remove polyps. Postprocedure instructions include maintaining an NPO (nothing by mouth) status until the sedation wears off and the client is alert, taking vital signs every 15 to 30 minutes until the client is alert, keeping side rails up until the client is stable, assessing for rectal bleeding and clots, and monitoring for manifestations of bowel perforation and hypovolemic shock. The client is told that fullness and mild abdominal cramping are expected for several hours.

Test-Taking Strategy: Focus on the subject, interventions in the immediate postprocedure plan. Recalling that the client receives sedation for this procedure and recalling the complications associated with this procedure will assist in answering the question. Also note the word *immediately* in option 6, the only incorrect option. Remember that fullness and mild abdominal cramping are expected for several hours after the procedure. Review nursing interventions following colonoscopy if you had difficulty with this question.

Level of Cognitive Ability: Application
Client Needs: Physiological Integrity
Integrated Process: Nursing Process/Planning
Content Area: Reduction of Risk Potential

Reference
Ignatavicius D, Workman M: *Medical surgical nursing: critical thinking for collaborative care,* ed 5, Philadelphia, 2006, Saunders, p 1245.

Multiple Response

171. The nurse provides information to a client with gastroesophageal reflux disease (GERD) about the factors that contribute to decreased lower esophageal sphincter (LES) pressure. The nurse tells the client that which factors contribute to decreased LES pressure? Select all that apply.

- ❏ **1** Alcohol
- ❏ **2** Fatty foods
- ❏ **3** Citrus fruits
- ❏ **4** Baked potatoes
- ❏ **5** Caffeinated beverages
- ❏ **6** Tomatoes and tomato products

Answer: 1, 2, 3, 5, 6

Rationale: GERD occurs as a result of the backward flow (reflux) of gastrointestinal contents into the esophagus. The most common cause of GERD is inappropriate relaxation of the LES, which allows the reflux of gastric contents into the esophagus and exposes the esophageal mucosa to gastric contents. Factors that influence the tone and contractility of the LES and lower LES pressure include fatty foods; caffeinated beverages such as coffee, tea, and cola; chocolate; citrus fruits; tomatoes and tomato products; nicotine in cigarette smoke; calcium channel blockers; nitrates; anticholinergics; high levels of estrogen and progesterone; peppermint and spearmint; alcohol; and nasogastric tube placement.

Test-Taking Strategy: Note the client's diagnosis and focus on the subject, factors that contribute to decreased LES pressure. Read each option and consider whether the item will aggravate the client's condition. The only item that will not is option 4, baked potatoes. Review the factors that contribute to decreased LES pressure if you had difficulty with this question.

Level of Cognitive Ability: Application
Client Needs: Physiological Integrity
Integrated Process: Nursing Process/Implementation
Content Area: Reduction of Risk Potential

Reference
Ignatavicius D, Workman M: *Medical surgical nursing: critical thinking for collaborative care,* ed 5, Philadelphia, 2006, Saunders, p 1261.

Multiple Response

172. The nurse provides a client with dietary information about measures to prevent dumping syndrome after a Billroth II procedure. Which instructions does the nurse give the client? Select all that apply.

❏ **1** Eat high-fiber foods.
❏ **2** Eat three large meals a day.
❏ **3** Drink liquids between meals only.
❏ **4** Eat foods that are high in carbohydrates.
❏ **5** Eat foods that are low in fat and protein.
❏ **6** Eliminate milk, sweets, and sugars from the diet.

Answer: 3, 6

Rationale: Dumping syndrome refers to a constellation of vasomotor symptoms after eating, especially after a Billroth II procedure. This syndrome occurs as a result of the rapid emptying of gastric contents into the small intestine, which shifts fluid into the gut, causing abdominal distention. Early manifestations, which typically occur 30 minutes after eating, include vertigo, tachycardia, syncope, sweating, pallor, palpitations, and the desire to lie down. General dietary measures include eating several small meals a day; eating foods that are high in fat and protein content and low in carbohydrate content; eating low-roughage foods; eliminating milk, sweets, and sugars from the diet; and drinking liquids between meals only.

Test-Taking Strategy: Focus on the client's diagnosis. Recall that dumping syndrome occurs as a result of the rapid emptying of gastric contents into the small intestine. Next read each option and think about how it may precipitate this response. Review dietary measures to prevent dumping syndrome if you had difficulty with this question.

Level of Cognitive Ability: Application
Client Needs: Physiological Integrity
Integrated Process: Teaching and Learning
Content Area: Reduction of Risk Potential

Reference
Ignatavicius D, Workman M: *Medical surgical nursing: critical thinking for collaborative care,* ed 5, Philadelphia, 2006, Saunders, p 1261.

Multiple Response

173. The nurse provides information to a client with a colostomy about the foods that will help prevent odor from the colostomy and tells the client to consume which foods? Select all that apply.

❑ **1** Parsley
❑ **2** Yogurt
❑ **3** Buttermilk
❑ **4** Cucumbers
❑ **5** Cauliflower
❑ **6** Cranberry juice

Answer: 1, 2, 3, 6

Rationale: The nurse should provide information about foods and measures that will prevent odor from a colostomy. Buttermilk, cranberry juice, parsley, and yogurt will prevent odor. Charcoal filters, pouch deodorizers, or placement of a breath mint in the pouch will eliminate odors. Foods that cause flatus and thus odor, including broccoli, Brussels sprouts, cabbage, cauliflower, cucumbers, mushrooms, and peas, should be avoided.

Test-Taking Strategy: Focus on the subject, foods to control odor. Eliminate options 4 and 5 using basic knowledge regarding nutrition, since these foods cause flatus. Review the foods to control odor in a client with a colostomy if you had difficulty with this question.

Level of Cognitive Ability: Application
Client Needs: Physiological Integrity
Integrated Process: Teaching and Learning
Content Area: Physiological Adaptation

Reference
Ignatavicius D, Workman M: *Medical surgical nursing: critical thinking for collaborative care,* ed 5, Philadelphia, 2006, Saunders, p 1325.

Multiple Response

174. A nurse is monitoring a client diagnosed with a ruptured appendix for signs of peritonitis and assesses for which of the following? Select all that apply.

❑ **1** Bradycardia
❑ **2** Distended abdomen
❑ **3** Subnormal temperature
❑ **4** Rigid, boardlike abdomen
❑ **5** Diminishing bowel sounds
❑ **6** Inability to pass flatus or feces

Answer: 2, 4, 5, 6

Rationale: Peritonitis is an acute inflammation of the visceral and parietal peritoneum, the endothelial lining of the abdominal cavity. Clinical manifestations include a rigid, boardlike abdomen; abdominal pain (localized, poorly localized, or referred to the shoulder or thorax); distended abdomen; anorexia, nausea, and vomiting; diminishing bowel sounds; inability to pass flatus or feces; rebound tenderness in the abdomen; high fever; tachycardia; dehydration from the high fever; decreased urinary output; hiccups; and possible compromise in respiratory status.

Test-Taking Strategy: Focus on the subject, signs of peritonitis. Remember that the suffix *-itis* indicates inflammation or infection. This will assist in determining that options 1 and 3 are incorrect. In inflammation the client would experience an elevated temperature, and tachycardia is a physiological bodily response to fever. Review the signs of peritonitis if you had difficulty with this question.

Level of Cognitive Ability: Analysis
Client Needs: Physiological Integrity
Integrated Process: Nursing Process/Assessment
Content Area: Physiological Adaptation

Reference
Ignatavicius D, Workman M: *Medical surgical nursing: critical thinking for collaborative care,* ed 5, Philadelphia, 2006, Saunders, p 1341.

Multiple Response

175. A client begins to experience a tonic-clonic seizure. The nurse takes which of the following actions? Select all that apply.

- ❑ 1 Restrain the client.
- ❑ 2 Turn the client to the side.
- ❑ 3 Maintain the client's airway.
- ❑ 4 Place a padded tongue blade into the client's mouth.
- ❑ 5 Loosen any restrictive clothing that the client is wearing.
- ❑ 6 Protect the client from injury, and guide the client's movements.

Answer: 2, 3, 5, 6

Rationale: Precautions are taken to prevent a client from sustaining injury during a seizure. The nurse would maintain the client's airway and turn the client to the side. The nurse would also protect the client from injury, guide the client's movements, and loosen any restrictive clothing. Restraints are never used because they could injure the client during the seizure. A padded tongue blade or any other object is never placed into the client's mouth after a seizure begins because the jaw may clench down.

Test-Taking Strategy: Focus on the subject, a client experiencing seizure activity. Visualize each of the actions to assist in answering correctly. Remember that restraints are never used because they could injure the client, and a padded tongue blade or any other object is never placed into the client's mouth. Review care of the client experiencing a seizure if you had difficulty with this question.

Level of Cognitive Ability: Application
Client Needs: Physiological Integrity
Integrated Process: Nursing Process/Implementation
Content Area: Physiological Adaptation

Reference
Ignatavicius D, Workman M: *Medical surgical nursing: critical thinking for collaborative care,* ed 5, Philadelphia, 2006, Saunders, p 953.

Multiple Response

176. A client is diagnosed with cholecystitis. The nurse reviews the client's medical record, expecting to note documentation of which manifestations of this disorder? Select all that apply.

❑ 1 Dyspepsia
❑ 2 Dark stools
❑ 3 Light-colored and clear urine
❑ 4 Feelings of abdominal fullness
❑ 5 Rebound tenderness in the abdomen
❑ 6 Upper abdominal pain that radiates to the right shoulder

Answer: 1, 4, 5, 6

Rationale: Cholecystitis is an inflammation of the gallbladder. Manifestations include upper abdominal pain or discomfort that can radiate to the right shoulder; pain triggered by a high-fat meal; anorexia, nausea, and vomiting; dyspepsia; eructation; flatulence; feelings of abdominal fullness; rebound tenderness (Blumberg's sign); fever; jaundice; and clay-colored stools, dark urine, and possible steatorrhea.

Test-Taking Strategy: Focus on the client's diagnosis and think about the pathophysiology associated with this disorder. This will assist in eliminating options 2 and 3. Remember that clay-colored stools and dark urine occur in this disorder. Review the manifestations of cholecystitis if you had difficulty with this question.

Level of Cognitive Ability: Analysis
Client Needs: Physiological Integrity
Integrated Process: Nursing Process/Assessment
Content Area: Physiological Adaptation

Reference
Ignatavicius D, Workman M: *Medical surgical nursing: critical thinking for collaborative care,* ed 5, Philadelphia, 2006, Saunders, p 1398.

Multiple Response

177. The nurse instructs a client with chronic pancreatitis about measures to prevent its exacerbation. The nurse provides the client with which information? Select all that apply.

   ❑ 1 Eat bland foods.
   ❑ 2 Avoid alcohol ingestion.
   ❑ 3 Avoid cigarette smoking.
   ❑ 4 Avoid caffeinated beverages.
   ❑ 5 Eat small meals and snacks high in calories.
   ❑ 6 Eat high-fat, low-protein, high-carbohydrate meals.

Answer: 1, 2, 3, 4, 5

Rationale: Chronic pancreatitis is a progressive, destructive disease of the pancreas, characterized by remissions and exacerbations (recurrence). Measures to prevent an exacerbation include avoiding caffeinated beverages, alcohol ingestion, and nicotine; eating bland, low-fat, high-protein, moderate-carbohydrate meals; avoiding gastric stimulants such as spices; and eating small meals and snacks high in calories.

Test-Taking Strategy: Focus on the subject, measures to prevent an exacerbation of chronic pancreatitis. Thinking about the pathophysiology associated with pancreatitis and noting the strategic words *high-fat* in option 6 will direct you to eliminate this option. Review the measures to prevent an exacerbation of chronic pancreatitis if you had difficulty with this question.

Level of Cognitive Ability: Application
Client Needs: Physiological Integrity
Integrated Process: Teaching and Learning
Content Area: Reduction of Risk Potential

Reference
Ignatavicius D, Workman M: *Medical surgical nursing: critical thinking for collaborative care,* ed 5, Philadelphia, 2006, Saunders, pp 1409, 1412.

Multiple Response

178. Which of the following are clinical manifestations of diabetes insipidus? Select all that apply.

❑ **1** Bradycardia
❑ **2** Hypertension
❑ **3** Poor skin turgor
❑ **4** Increased urinary output
❑ **5** Dry mucous membranes
❑ **6** Decreased pulse pressure

Answer: 3, 4, 5, 6

Rationale: Diabetes insipidus is a water metabolism problem caused by an antidiuretic hormone (ADH) deficiency (either a decrease in ADH synthesis or an inability of the kidneys to respond to ADH). Clinical manifestations include hypotension, decreased pulse pressure, tachycardia, weak peripheral pulses, increased urinary output, poor skin turgor, dry mucous membranes, and increased thirst.

Test-Taking Strategy: Focus on the client's diagnosis. Think about the pathophysiology of this disorder and recall that diabetes insipidus is caused by an ADH deficiency. This will assist in eliminating options 1 and 2. Review the manifestations of diabetes insipidus if you had difficulty with this question.

Level of Cognitive Ability: Analysis
Client Needs: Physiological Integrity
Integrated Process: Nursing Process/Assessment
Content Area: Physiological Adaptation

Reference

Ignatavicius D, Workman M: *Medical surgical nursing: critical thinking for collaborative care,* ed 5, Philadelphia, 2006, Saunders, p 1466.

Multiple Response

179. A client is diagnosed with hypothyroidism. The nurse performs an assessment on the client, expecting to note which findings? Select all that apply.

❑ **1** Weight loss
❑ **2** Bradycardia
❑ **3** Hypotension
❑ **4** Dry, scaly skin
❑ **5** Heat intolerance
❑ **6** Decreased body temperature

Answer: 2, 3, 4, 6

Rationale: The manifestations of hypothyroidism are the result of decreased metabolism from low levels of thyroid hormones. Some of these manifestations are cool, dry, scaly skin; dry, coarse, brittle hair; decreased hair growth; bradycardia; hypotension; decreased body temperature; cold intolerance; slowing of intellectual functioning; lethargy; weight gain; and constipation.

Test-Taking Strategy: Focus on the client's diagnosis and recall that hypothyroidism occurs as the result of decreased metabolism from low levels of thyroid hormones. Correlate *hypo*thyroidism with *decreased* body functioning to assist in answering the question. Weight loss and heat intolerance occur in hyperthyroidism. Review the manifestations of hypothyroidism if you had difficulty with this question.

Level of Cognitive Ability: Analysis
Client Needs: Physiological Integrity
Integrated Process: Nursing Process/Assessment
Content Area: Physiological Adaptation

Reference
Ignatavicius D, Workman M: *Medical surgical nursing: critical thinking for collaborative care,* ed 5, Philadelphia, 2006, Saunders, p 1488.

Multiple Response

180. The nurse provides information to a client with diabetes mellitus who is taking insulin about the signs of hypoglycemia. Which of the following signs should the nurse include in the information? Select all that apply.

- ❑ **1** Hunger
- ❑ **2** Sweating
- ❑ **3** Weakness
- ❑ **4** Nervousness
- ❑ **5** Cool clammy skin
- ❑ **6** Increased urinary output

Answer: 1, 2, 3, 4, 5

Rationale: Hypoglycemia is characterized by a blood glucose level of 50 mg/dL or below. Clinical manifestations of hypoglycemia include cool clammy skin, hunger, weakness, sweating, nervousness, blurred vision or double vision, tachycardia, and palpitations. Increased urinary output is a manifestation of hyperglycemia.

Test-Taking Strategy: Focus on the subject, the manifestations of hypoglycemia. Recall that hypoglycemia is characterized by a blood glucose level of 50 mg/dL or below. Next think about the manifestations that occur when the blood glucose level is low. Also recalling the 3 Ps associated with hyperglycemia—polyuria, polydipsia, and polyphagia—will assist in eliminating option 6. Review the manifestations associated with hypoglycemia and hyperglycemia if you had difficulty with this question.

Level of Cognitive Ability: Analysis
Client Needs: Physiological Integrity
Integrated Process: Teaching and Learning
Content Area: Physiological Adaptation

Reference
Ignatavicius D, Workman M: *Medical surgical nursing: critical thinking for collaborative care,* ed 5, Philadelphia, 2006, Saunders, p 1541.

Multiple Response

181. A client with calcium oxalate renal calculi is told to limit dietary intake of oxalate. The nurse provides the client with a list of foods high in oxalate and places which items on the list? Select all that apply.

❑ **1** Beets
❑ **2** Spinach
❑ **3** Rhubarb
❑ **4** Black tea
❑ **5** Chocolate
❑ **6** Watermelon

Answer: 1, 2, 3, 4, 5

Rationale: Food items that are high in oxalate include spinach, black tea, rhubarb, Swiss chard, cocoa, beets, wheat germ, pecans, peanuts, okra, chocolate, and lime peel.

Test-Taking Strategy: Knowledge regarding food items high in oxalate is needed to answer this question. Remembering that fruits are generally not sources of dietary oxalate will assist in answering questions similar to this one. Review the foods high in oxalate if you had difficulty with this question.

Level of Cognitive Ability: Application
Client Needs: Physiological Integrity
Integrated Process: Teaching and Learning
Content Area: Reduction of Risk Potential

Reference
Ignatavicius D, Workman M: *Medical surgical nursing: critical thinking for collaborative care,* ed 5, Philadelphia, 2006, Saunders, p 1697.

Multiple Response

182. The nurse prepares a care plan for a client receiving hemodialysis who has an arteriovenous (AV) fistula in the right arm. The nurse includes which interventions in the plan to ensure protecting the AV fistula? Select all that apply.

❑ **1** Assess pulses and circulation proximal to the fistula.

❑ **2** Palpate for thrills and auscultate for a bruit every 4 hours.

❑ **3** Check for bleeding and infection at hemodialysis needle insertion sites.

❑ **4** Avoid taking blood pressure or performing venipunctures in the extremity.

❑ **5** Instruct the client not to carry heavy objects or anything that compresses the extremity.

❑ **6** Instruct the client not to sleep in a position that places his or her body weight on top of the extremity.

Answer: 2, 3, 4, 5, 6

Rationale: An AV fistula is an internal anastomosis of an artery to a vein and is used as an access for hemodialysis. The nurse should implement the following to protect the fistula: avoid taking blood pressures or performing venipunctures in the extremity, palpate for thrills and auscultate for a bruit every 4 hours, assess pulses and circulation distal to the fistula, check for bleeding and infection at hemodialysis needle insertion sites, instruct the client not to carry heavy objects or anything that compresses the extremity, and instruct the client not to sleep in a position that places his or her body weight on top of the extremity.

Test-Taking Strategy: Focus on the subject, protecting the AV fistula. Visualize this vascular access device and read each option carefully. Noting the word *proximal* in option 1 will assist in eliminating this option. Review measures to protect an AV fistula if you had difficulty with this question.

Level of Cognitive Ability: Application
Client Needs: Physiological Integrity
Integrated Process: Nursing Process/Planning
Content Area: Reduction of Risk Potential

Reference
Ignatavicius D, Workman M: *Medical surgical nursing: critical thinking for collaborative care,* ed 5, Philadelphia, 2006, Saunders, p 1754.

Multiple Response

183. A child is admitted to the hospital with a diagnosis of nephrotic syndrome. The nurse reads the child's medical record and expects to note documentation of which manifestations of this disorder? Select all that apply.

❑ **1** Edema
❑ **2** Proteinuria
❑ **3** Hypertension
❑ **4** Abdominal pain
❑ **5** Increased weight
❑ **6** Hypoalbuminemia

Answer: 1, 2, 4, 5, 6

Rationale: Nephrotic syndrome refers to a kidney disorder characterized by proteinuria, hypoalbuminemia, and edema. The child also experiences anorexia, fatigue, abdominal pain, respiratory infection, and increased weight. The child's blood pressure is usually normal.

Test-Taking Strategy: Recalling that nephrotic syndrome is characterized by proteinuria, hypoalbuminemia, and edema will assist in determining the correct options. Also remember that the blood pressure is usually normal in this condition. Review the manifestations of nephrotic syndrome if you had difficulty with this question.

Level of Cognitive Ability: Analysis
Client Needs: Physiological Integrity
Integrated Process: Nursing Process/Assessment
Content Area: Physiological Adaptation

Reference
McKinney E, James S, Murray S, et al: *Maternal-child nursing,* ed 2, Philadelphia, 2005, Saunders, p 1175.

Multiple Response

184. The nurse instructs a mother of a child who had a plaster cast applied to the arm about measures that will help the cast dry. Which instructions should the nurse provide to the mother? Select all that apply.

❏ **1** Lift the cast using the fingertips.
❏ **2** Place the child on a firm mattress.
❏ **3** Direct a fan toward the cast to facilitate drying.
❏ **4** Support the cast and adjacent joints with pillows.
❏ **5** Place the extremity with the cast in a dependent position.
❏ **6** Reposition the extremity with the cast every 2 to 4 hours.

Answer: 2, 3, 4, 6

Rationale: To help the cast dry, the child should be placed on a firm mattress. The cast and adjacent joints should be elevated and supported with pillows. To ensure thorough drying, the extremity with the cast should be repositioned every 2 to 4 hours. The cast is lifted by using the palms of the hands (not the fingertips) to prevent indentation in the wet cast surface. Indentations could possibly cause pressure on the skin under the cast. A fan may be directed toward the cast to facilitate drying. Once the cast is dry, the cast should sound hollow and be cool to touch.

Test-Taking Strategy: Focus on the subject, measures that will help the cast dry. Eliminate option 1 because of the word *fingertips* and option 5 because of the word *dependent*. Review measures that will help a cast dry if you had difficulty with this question.

Level of Cognitive Ability: Application
Client Needs: Physiological Integrity
Integrated Process: Teaching and Learning
Content Area: Reduction of Risk Potential

Reference
Ignatavicius D, Workman M: *Medical surgical nursing: critical thinking for collaborative care,* ed 5, Philadelphia, 2006, Saunders, pp 1199-1200.

Multiple Response

185. The nurse provides activity instructions to a client who had a total abdominal hysterectomy. The nurse provides which instructions to the client? Select all that apply.

- ❑ 1 Sit as much as possible.
- ❑ 2 Take baths rather than showers.
- ❑ 3 Limit stair climbing to five times a day.
- ❑ 4 Avoid lifting anything heavier than 5 pounds.
- ❑ 5 Gradually increase walking as exercise but stop before becoming fatigued.
- ❑ 6 Avoid jogging, aerobic exercises, sports, or any strenuous exercise for 6 weeks.

Answer: 3, 4, 5, 6

Rationale: After a total abdominal hysterectomy, the client should limit stair climbing to five times a day. The client should also take showers rather than tub baths. Additional instructions include avoiding lifting anything heavier than 5 pounds; walking indoors for the first week and then gradually increasing walking as exercise, but stopping before becoming fatigued; avoiding the sitting position for extended periods; avoiding crossing the legs at the knees; avoiding jogging, aerobic exercises, sports, or any strenuous exercise for 6 weeks; and avoiding driving for at least 4 weeks or until the surgeon has given permission to do so.

Test-Taking Strategy: Read each option carefully, focusing on the type and location of the surgery and the importance of protecting the surgical area. This will assist in eliminating options 1 and 2. Review activity instructions following total abdominal hysterectomy if you had difficulty with this question.

Level of Cognitive Ability: Application
Client Needs: Physiological Integrity
Integrated Process: Teaching and Learning
Content Area: Reduction of Risk Potential

Reference
Ignatavicius D, Workman M: *Medical surgical nursing: critical thinking for collaborative care,* ed 5, Philadelphia, 2006, Saunders, p 1841.

Multiple Response

186. A client has a total serum calcium level of 7.5 mg/dL. Which clinical manifestations would the nurse expect to note on assessment of the client? Select all that apply.

❑ 1 Constipation
❑ 2 Muscle twitches
❑ 3 Hypoactive bowel sounds
❑ 4 Hyperactive deep tendon reflexes
❑ 5 Positive Trousseau's sign and positive Chvostek's sign
❑ 6 Prolonged ST interval and QT interval on electrocardiogram (ECG)

Answer: 2, 4, 5, 6

Rationale: Hypocalcemia is a total serum calcium level below 9.0 mg/dL. Clinical manifestations of hypocalcemia include decreased heart rate, diminished peripheral pulses, hypotension, and prolonged ST interval and QT interval on ECG. Neuromuscular manifestations include anxiety and irritability; paresthesia followed by numbness; muscle twitches, cramps, tetany, and seizures; hyperactive deep tendon reflexes; and positive Trousseau's sign and Chvostek's sign. Gastrointestinal manifestations include increased gastric motility, hyperactive bowel sounds, abdominal cramping, and diarrhea.

Test-Taking Strategy: Note the data in the question and the calcium level. First determine that the level is low and the client is experiencing hypocalcemia. Next think about the manifestations associated with hypocalcemia. Remember that hyperactive bowel sounds and diarrhea occur in hypocalcemia. Review the manifestations of hypocalcemia if you had difficulty with this question.

Level of Cognitive Ability: Analysis
Client Needs: Physiological Integrity
Integrated Process: Nursing Process/Assessment
Content Area: Physiological Adaptation

Reference
Ignatavicius D, Workman M: *Medical surgical nursing: critical thinking for collaborative care,* ed 5, Philadelphia, 2006, Saunders, p 238.

Multiple Response

187. Which of the following are signs and symptoms of infiltration at the catheter site of an intravenous (IV) infusion? Select all that apply.

- ❑ **1** Slowing of the IV rate
- ❑ **2** Tenderness at the insertion site
- ❑ **3** Edema around the insertion site
- ❑ **4** Skin tightness at the insertion site
- ❑ **5** Fluid leaking from the insertion site
- ❑ **6** Warmth of skin at the insertion site

Answer: 1, 2, 3, 4, 5

Rationale: Infiltration is the leakage of an IV solution into the extravascular tissue. Signs and symptoms include slowing of the IV rate; increasing edema in or around the catheter insertion site; complaints of skin tightness, burning, tenderness, or general discomfort at the insertion site; blanching or coolness of the skin; and fluid leaking from the insertion site.

Test-Taking Strategy: Focus on the data in the question. Read each option, thinking about the characteristics of infiltration. Recalling that infiltration is the leakage of an IV solution into the extravascular tissue will assist in eliminating option 6. Remember that fluid infusing into tissue will result in coolness, not warmth. Review the signs and symptoms of infiltration if you had difficulty with this question.

Level of Cognitive Ability: Analysis
Client Needs: Physiological Integrity
Integrated Process: Nursing Process/Assessment
Content Area: Physiological Adaptation

Reference

Ignatavicius D, Workman M: *Medical surgical nursing: critical thinking for collaborative care,* ed 5, Philadelphia, 2006, Saunders, p 259.

Multiple Response

188. The nurse provides which medication instructions to a client who has been prescribed levothyroxine (Synthroid)? Select all that apply.

- ❏ **1** Monitor your own pulse rate.
- ❏ **2** Take the medication in the morning.
- ❏ **3** Notify the physician if chest pain occurs.
- ❏ **4** Take the medication at the same time each day.
- ❏ **5** Expect the pulse rate to be greater than 100 beats/min.
- ❏ **6** It may take 1 to 3 weeks for a full therapeutic effect to occur.

Answer: 1, 2, 3, 4, 6

Rationale: Levothyroxine is a thyroid hormone. The client is instructed to take the medication at the same time each day to maintain hormone levels. The client is also instructed to take the medication in the morning before breakfast to prevent insomnia. The client is told not to discontinue the medication and that thyroid replacement is lifelong. Additional instructions include monitoring own pulse rate and contacting the physician if the rate is greater than 100 beats/min; and notifying the physician if chest pain occurs, or if weight loss, nervousness and tremors, or insomnia develops. The client is also told that full therapeutic effect may take 1 to 3 weeks and that he or she needs to have follow-up thyroid blood studies to monitor therapy.

Test-Taking Strategy: Focus on the medication name and recall that levothyroxine is a thyroid hormone to treat hypothyroidism. Think about the effects of the medication as you read each option. Noting the words *greater than 100 beats/min* in option 5 will assist in eliminating this option. Review client teaching points related to levothyroxine if you had difficulty with this question.

Level of Cognitive Ability: Application
Client Needs: Physiological Integrity
Integrated Process: Teaching and Learning
Content Area: Pharmacological and Parenteral Therapies

Reference
Hodgson B, Kizior R: *Saunders nursing drug handbook 2007*, Philadelphia, 2007, Saunders, pp 686-688.

Multiple Response

189. A client taking warfarin sodium (Coumadin) has been instructed to limit the intake of foods high in vitamin K. The nurse instructs the client to avoid which food items? Select all that apply.

❑ 1 Tea
❑ 2 Turnips
❑ 3 Oranges
❑ 4 Cabbage
❑ 5 Broccoli
❑ 6 Strawberries

Answer: 1, 2, 4, 5

Rationale: Warfarin sodium is an anticoagulant that interferes with the hepatic synthesis of vitamin K–dependent clotting factors. The client is instructed to limit the intake of foods high in vitamin K while taking this medication. These foods include broccoli, cabbage, turnips, greens, fish, liver, and coffee or tea (caffeine). Oranges and strawberries are high in vitamin C.

Test-Taking Strategy: Knowledge regarding the foods high in vitamin K is needed to answer correctly. However, note that options 3 and 6 are alike in that they are both fruits. Review the foods high in vitamin K if you had difficulty with this question.

Level of Cognitive Ability: Application
Client Needs: Physiological Integrity
Integrated Process: Teaching and Learning
Content Area: Pharmacological and Parenteral Therapies

References
Black J, Hawks J: *Medical-surgical nursing: clinical management for positive outcomes,* ed 7, Philadelphia, 2005, Saunders, p 670.
Hodgson B, Kizior R: *Saunders nursing drug handbook 2007,* Philadelphia, 2007, Saunders, pp 1221-1222.

Multiple Response

190. The nurse performs an assessment on a client newly diagnosed with rheumatoid arthritis. The nurse expects to note which early manifestations of the disease? Select all that apply.

❏ **1** Fatigue
❏ **2** Anorexia
❏ **3** Weakness
❏ **4** Low-grade fever
❏ **5** Joint deformities
❏ **6** Joint inflammation

Answer: 1, 2, 3, 4, 6

Rationale: Rheumatoid arthritis is a chronic, progressive, systemic inflammatory autoimmune disease process that primarily affects the synovial joints. It also affects other joints and body tissues. Early manifestations include joint inflammation, low-grade fever, fatigue, weakness, anorexia, and paresthesia. Joint deformities are late manifestations.

Test-Taking Strategy: Focus on the data in the question and note the strategic word *early.* Keeping this word in mind will assist in eliminating option 5, since joint deformities are late manifestations. Review the early and late manifestations of rheumatoid arthritis if you had difficulty with this question.

Level of Cognitive Ability: Analysis
Client Needs: Physiological Integrity
Integrated Process: Nursing Process/Assessment
Content Area: Physiological Adaptation

Reference
Ignatavicius D, Workman M: *Medical surgical nursing: critical thinking for collaborative care,* ed 5, Philadelphia, 2006, Saunders, p 394.

REFERENCES

Black J, Hawks J: *Medical-surgical nursing: clinical management for positive outcomes,* ed 7, Philadelphia, 2005, Saunders.

Chernecky C, Berger B: *Laboratory tests and diagnostic procedures,* ed 4, Philadelphia, 2004, Saunders.

Harkreader H, Hogan MA: *Fundamentals of nursing: caring and clinical judgment,* ed 2, Philadelphia, 2004, Saunders.

Hodgson B, Kizior R: *Saunders nursing drug handbook 2007,* Philadelphia, 2007, Saunders.

Ignatavicius D, Workman M: *Medical surgical nursing: critical thinking for collaborative care,* ed 5, Philadelphia, 2006, Saunders.

Kee J, Hayes E: *Pharmacology: a nursing process approach,* ed 5, St Louis, 2006, Mosby.

Kee J, Marshall S: *Clinical calculations: with applications to general and specialty areas,* ed 5, Philadelphia, 2004, Saunders.

Macklin D, Chernecky C, Infortuna H: *Math for clinical practice,* St Louis, 2005, Mosby.

McKinney E, James S, Murray S, et al: *Maternal-child nursing,* ed 2, Philadelphia, 2005, Saunders.

Mosby's medical, nursing, and allied health dictionary, ed 6, St Louis, 2006, Mosby.

National Council of State Boards of Nursing: www.ncsbn.org.

National Council of State Boards of Nursing: *National Council of State Boards of Nursing Test Plan for the NCLEX-RN® Examination* (effective date: April 2007), Chicago, 2006, The Council.

Potter P, Perry A: *Fundamentals of nursing,* ed 6, St Louis, 2005, Mosby.

Varcarolis E, Carson V, Shoemaker N: *Foundations of psychiatric mental health nursing,* ed 5, Philadelphia, 2006, Saunders.

Wilson S, Giddens J: *Health assessment for nursing practice,* ed 3, St Louis, 2005, Mosby.

Wong D, Perry S, Hockenberry M, et al: *Maternal child nursing care,* ed 3, St Louis, 2006, Mosby.

Comprehensive Test

Multiple Response

191. A nurse is developing a postprocedure care plan for a client who is going to have a lumbar puncture (spinal tap). Which of the following interventions should be included in the care plan? Select all that apply.

❏ 1 Increase fluid intake.
❏ 2 Administer analgesics for headache, if it occurs.
❏ 3 Maintain an NPO status until a gag reflex returns.
❏ 4 Maintain bed rest in a flat position for 4 to 8 hours.
❏ 5 Assess the client for decreasing level of consciousness.
❏ 6 Encourage deep breathing and coughing every 30 minutes.

Answer: 1, 2, 4, 5

Rationale: A lumbar puncture is the insertion of a needle into the subarachnoid space and is done to obtain pressure readings, obtain cerebrospinal fluid (CSF) for analysis, check for spinal blockage, inject contrast medium or air for diagnostic study, inject spinal anesthetics or certain other medications, or reduce mild to moderate increased intracranial pressure (ICP) in certain conditions. After a lumbar puncture the client is generally restricted to bed rest in a flat position for 4 to 8 hours as prescribed by the physician or as determined by hospital policy. This prevents CSF leakage from the puncture site. Fluid intake is increased (to 3000 mL unless contraindicated) for 24 to 48 hours to facilitate CSF production. The client can eat and drink as before the test. The client's neurological status is monitored, especially if the lumbar puncture was performed to reduce ICP. Analgesics are administered for a headache, if it occurs. It is not necessary to encourage deep breathing and coughing every 30 minutes.

Test-Taking Strategy: Focus on the subject, a lumbar puncture. Think about the purpose and visualize the procedure for this test as you read each of the options. This will assist in answering correctly. Review this procedure if you had difficulty with this question.

Level of Cognitive Ability: Application
Client Needs: Physiological Integrity
Integrated Process: Nursing Process/Planning
Content Area: Reduction of Risk Potential

Reference
Ignatavicius D, Workman M: *Medical surgical nursing: critical thinking for collaborative care,* ed 5, Philadelphia, 2006, Saunders, p 942.

Multiple Response

192. A nurse is preparing a care plan for a client diagnosed with epilepsy. Which of the following nursing diagnoses may apply to this client? Select all that apply.

❏ 1 Chronic Confusion related to epilepsy

❏ 2 Risk for Falls related to impaired balance

❏ 3 Risk for Ineffective Breathing pattern related to neuromuscular dysfunction

❏ 4 Deficient Diversional Activity related to inability to participate in social functions

❏ 5 Disturbed Sleep Pattern related to changes in sleep phases, anxiety, or depression

❏ 6 Ineffective Coping related to uncertainty and perception of inadequate level of control

Answer: 2, 3, 6

Rationale: Epilepsy is a chronic disorder characterized by recurrent, unprovoked seizure activity. Nursing diagnoses that may apply to clients with epilepsy include Risk for Falls related to impaired balance, Risk for Ineffective Breathing Pattern related to neuromuscular dysfunction, and Ineffective Coping related to uncertainty and perception of inadequate level of control. Chronic confusion is not a characteristic of epilepsy. The client with epilepsy is able to participate in social functions. Disturbed sleep pattern related to changes in sleep phases, anxiety, or depression is not associated with epilepsy.

Test-Taking Strategy: Focus on the client's diagnosis. Think about the description and pathophysiology associated with this condition. Visualize each of the options in terms of its pathophysiology to answer correctly. Review this disorder if you had difficulty with this question.

Level of Cognitive Ability: Analysis
Client Needs: Physiological Integrity
Integrated Process: Nursing Process/Analysis
Content Area: Physiological Adaptation

Reference
Ignatavicius D, Workman M: *Medical surgical nursing: critical thinking for collaborative care,* ed 5, Philadelphia, 2006, Saunders, p 951.

Multiple Response

193. The nurse should implement which measures to prevent infection in a hospitalized immunocompromised client? Select all that apply.

    ❑ 1 Use strict aseptic technique for all invasive procedures.
    ❑ 2 Insert a Foley catheter to eliminate the need to use a bedpan.
    ❑ 3 Use good hand-washing technique before touching the client.
    ❑ 4 Keep fresh flowers and potted plants out of the client's room.
    ❑ 5 Place the client in a semiprivate room with another client who is immunocompromised.
    ❑ 6 Keep frequently used equipment such as a blood pressure cuff in the client's room for use by the client only.

Answer: 1, 3, 4, 6

Rationale: An immunocompromised client is at high risk for infection, and specific measures are taken to prevent infection. The client is placed in a private room. Good hand-washing technique is used before touching the client. Strict aseptic technique is necessary for all invasive procedures; however, invasive procedures are avoided as much as possible. Foley catheters are avoided because of the risk of infection associated with their use. Fresh fruits, fresh flowers, and potted plants are kept out of the client's room because they harbor organisms, placing the client at risk for infection. Frequently used equipment such as a blood pressure cuff, stethoscope, or thermometer is kept in the client's room for use by the client only. The client is also monitored daily for any signs of infection.

Test-Taking Strategy: Focus on the subject, measures to prevent infection. Eliminate option 2, recalling that infection is associated with the use of a Foley catheter. Next eliminate option 5 because of the words *semiprivate room*. Review measures to prevent infection in a hospitalized immunocompromised client if you had difficulty with this question.

Level of Cognitive Ability: Application
Client Needs: Safe and Effective Care Environment
Integrated Process: Nursing Process/Implementation
Content Area: Safety and Infection Control

Reference
Ignatavicius D, Workman M: *Medical surgical nursing: critical thinking for collaborative care,* ed 5, Philadelphia, 2006, Saunders, p 438.

Multiple Response

194. The nurse is caring for a client who underwent reconstructive plastic surgery and has a musculocutaneous flap at the deltopectoral area. Which of the following clinical manifestations would the nurse report immediately to the physician? Select all that apply.

- ❑ 1 Pallor in the flap
- ❑ 2 Duskiness in the flap
- ❑ 3 Warm skin at the flap site
- ❑ 4 Increasing pain in the flap
- ❑ 5 Capillary refill of 3 seconds in the flap
- ❑ 6 Weak but regular pulses distal to the flap site

Answer: 1, 2, 4

Rationale: Skin flaps are sections of skin rotated from their origin to cover a defect. A deltopectoral flap is a skin flap to reconstruct a neck after excision of cancer. Flaps composed of both muscle and skin are called musculocutaneous flaps. An expected outcome is that the client will maintain effective peripheral perfusion, and the nurse monitors closely for signs of impairment. Signs of impairment that the nurse needs to report to the physician immediately include development of coolness in the flap, duskiness or pallor, slowing of capillary refill, loss of pulses, and increasing pain in the flap.

Test-Taking Strategy: Focus on the subject of the question, signs of ineffective peripheral perfusion. Recall these signs and select option 1 because of the word *pallor*, option 2 because of the word *duskiness,* and option 4 because of the words *increasing pain.* Review the signs of ineffective peripheral perfusion if you had difficulty with this question.

Level of Cognitive Ability: Analysis
Client Needs: Physiological Integrity
Integrated Process: Nursing Process/Assessment
Content Area: Physiological Adaptation

Reference
Black J, Hawks J: *Medical-surgical nursing: clinical management for positive outcomes,* ed 7, Philadelphia, 2005, Saunders, pp 1427-1428.

Multiple Response

195. The emergency department nurse is assessing a client with an inhalation burn injury for manifestations of carbon monoxide (CO) poisoning. Which of the following would the nurse expect to note? Select all that apply.

❑ **1** Bradypnea
❑ **2** Bradycardia
❑ **3** Impaired visual acuity
❑ **4** Flushing and headache
❑ **5** Nausea and impaired dexterity
❑ **6** Vomiting, dizziness, and syncope

Answer: 3, 4, 5, 6

Rationale: CO poisoning is a toxic condition in which carbon monoxide gas has been inhaled and binds to hemoglobin molecules, thus displacing oxygen from the red blood cells and decreasing the oxygen-carrying capacity of the blood. The clinical manifestations of acute CO poisoning are directly related to the level of carboxyhemoglobin saturation and relative degree of tissue hypoxia. Initial manifestations are related to decreased cerebral tissue oxygenation and are neurological in nature. Clinical manifestations include impaired visual acuity (5% to 10% CO level); flushing and headache (11% to 20% CO level); nausea and impaired dexterity (21% to 30% CO level); vomiting, dizziness, and syncope (31% to 40% CO level); tachypnea and tachycardia (41% to 50% CO level); and coma and death (greater than 50% CO level).

Test-Taking Strategy: Focus on the subject, the manifestations of CO poisoning. Note that the client had experienced an inhalation burn injury, and recall the physiological response of a client with this type of injury and with CO poisoning. This will assist in eliminating options 1 and 2. Review the manifestations of CO poisoning if you had difficulty with this question.

Level of Cognitive Ability: Analysis
Client Needs: Physiological Integrity
Integrated Process: Nursing Process/Assessment
Content Area: Physiological Adaptation

References
Black J, Hawks J: *Medical-surgical nursing: clinical management for positive outcomes,* ed 7, Philadelphia, 2005, Saunders, p 1440.
Mosby's medical, nursing, and allied health dictionary, ed 7, St Louis, 2006, Mosby, p 297.

Multiple Response

196. A nurse develops a care plan for a client receiving heparin sodium. The nurse includes which interventions in the care plan? Select all that apply.

❑ **1** Provide the client with a soft toothbrush.

❑ **2** Monitor the client for bruising and bleeding.

❑ **3** Have the antidote (protamine sulfate) available.

❑ **4** Apply pressure to venipuncture and other injection sites.

❑ **5** Allow the client to take acetylsalicylic acid (aspirin) for headache.

❑ **6** Allow the client to use a straight razor for shaving with supervision.

Answer: 1, 2, 3, 4

Rationale: Heparin sodium is an anticoagulant, and measures are implemented to monitor for and prevent bleeding. These include monitoring the client for bruising or bleeding; avoiding puncture sites and applying pressure to venipuncture and other injection sites; and avoiding the use of firm toothbrushes, straight razors, and rectal thermometers. The antidote for heparin sodium (protamine sulfate) should be available in the event of bleeding. Salicylates such as acetylsalicylic acid are avoided because they can increase the anticoagulation effect.

Test-Taking Strategy: Focus on the name of the medication. Recall that heparin sodium is an anticoagulant and that the primary concern is bleeding. Read each option, thinking about its effect on bleeding. This will assist in answering correctly. Also remember that the antidote for heparin sodium is protamine sulfate. Review nursing interventions for the client receiving heparin sodium if you had difficulty with this question.

Level of Cognitive Ability: Application
Client Needs: Physiological Integrity
Integrated Process: Nursing Process/Planning
Content Area: Pharmacological and Parenteral Therapies

Reference
Ignatavicius D, Workman M: *Medical surgical nursing: critical thinking for collaborative care,* ed 5, Philadelphia, 2006, Saunders, p 653.

Multiple Response

197. A nurse is assessing a client who has chronic arterial insufficiency of the lower extremities. Which of the following clinical manifestations would the nurse expect the client to exhibit? Select all that apply.

- ❑ **1** Warm skin temperature
- ❑ **2** Intermittent claudication
- ❑ **3** Thin, shiny, hairless skin
- ❑ **4** Pale skin with dependent rubor
- ❑ **5** Decreased to absent pulses in the affected extremity
- ❑ **6** Pain that decreases when the legs are elevated above heart level

Answer: 2, 3, 4, 5

Rationale: Arterial insufficiency of the lower extremities is characterized by hardening, thickening, and loss of elasticity of the walls of the arteries in the legs. Chronic arterial insufficiency produces decreased or absent arterial pulses; thin, shiny, hairless skin; thick, ridged toenails; cool skin temperature; pain with ambulation (intermittent claudication); pain that may worsen with leg elevation or at night; and skin that is pale when the legs are elevated above heart level and dusky red after they are placed in a dependent position (dependent rubor). Edema is not usually present in pure arterial insufficiency. There may be ulcers from trauma over pressure points or on the tips of the toes.

Test-Taking Strategy: Focus on the subject, the manifestations of chronic arterial insufficiency of the lower extremities. The strategic word in this question is *arterial.* Think about the anatomy and physiology of and the blood flow direction in the arterial system to assist in answering the question. Remember that in arterial disease the skin temperature is cool and pain increases when the legs are elevated above heart level. Review the manifestations of both arterial and venous insufficiency if you had difficulty with this question.

Level of Cognitive Ability: Analysis
Client Needs: Physiological Integrity
Integrated Process: Nursing Process/Assessment
Content Area: Physiological Adaptation

Reference
Black J, Hawks J: *Medical-surgical nursing: clinical management for positive outcomes,* ed 7, Philadelphia, 2005, Saunders, pp 1477-1478.

Multiple Response

198. The nurse is caring for a client following contrast angiography with a transaxillary approach. The nurse expects to note which routine postprocedural orders documented in the client's record? Select all that apply.

- ❏ **1** Bed rest for 6 to 8 hours
- ❏ **2** Resumption of preprocedure diet and medications
- ❏ **3** Maintenance of the punctured extremity in straight alignment
- ❏ **4** Continuous hydration intravenously and orally for 6 to 8 hours
- ❏ **5** Monitoring of vital signs, distal pulses, and the site for hematoma formation
- ❏ **6** Assessment of blood urea nitrogen (BUN) and creatinine levels on the following day

Answer: 2, 3, 4, 5, 6

Rationale: Contrast angiography is an invasive procedure that involves injecting a contrast agent into the arterial system and performing radiographic studies. Nursing care after angiography usually involves routine postprocedural orders, including frequent assessment of vital signs, neurological function, and distal pulses, with particular attention to the extremity that has been punctured; assessment of the puncture site for hematoma (bruising) and of the appearance of the extremity distal to the puncture site; bed rest for 6 to 8 hours for a transfemoral approach (however, a transaxillary approach does not require postprocedure bed rest), with the punctured extremity kept in straight alignment; encouragement of oral fluid intake and continuous intravenous hydration for 6 to 8 hours to assist with contrast excretion; assessment of the BUN and creatinine levels the following day (contrast material can be nephrotoxic); and the resumption of preprocedure diet and medications. If the client was receiving heparin or another anticoagulant, its administration may not be resumed until sealing of the punctured site has been confirmed.

Test-Taking Strategy: Note the strategic words *transaxillary approach*. This will assist in determining that bed rest is unnecessary. Next, use of the ABCs, airway, breathing, and circulation, will assist in determining that monitoring vital signs, distal pulses, and the site for hematoma formation is a correct intervention. Finally, knowledge of the general care for a client after angiography aids in selecting the remaining options. Review care for a client after contrast angiography via a transaxillary approach if you had difficulty with this question.

Level of Cognitive Ability: Analysis
Client Needs: Physiological Integrity
Integrated Process: Nursing Process/Analysis
Content Area: Reduction of Risk Potential

Reference
Black J, Hawks J: *Medical-surgical nursing: clinical management for positive outcomes,* ed 7, Philadelphia, 2005, Saunders, p 1486.

Multiple Response

199. The nurse is conducting a physical assessment on a client with hypertension. To assess the status of target organs affected by hypertension, the nurse should do which of the following? Select all that apply.

❏ **1** Examine the neck.
❏ **2** Auscultate the heart.
❏ **3** Auscultate the lungs.
❏ **4** Examine the extremities.
❏ **5** Examine neurological function.
❏ **6** Examine the eye (funduscopic examination).

Answer: 1, 2, 4, 5, 6

Rationale: Target organs affected by hypertension include the heart and blood vessels, eyes, brain, and kidneys. Physical assessment of a client with hypertension should include assessment of vital signs and weight and a funduscopic examination of the eyes, looking for retinal arteriolar narrowing, hemorrhages, exudates, and papilledema. The nurse should also examine the neck for distended veins and auscultate for carotid bruits; auscultate the heart for increased heart rate and dysrhythmias; examine and auscultate the abdomen for bruits, aortic dilation, and enlarged kidneys; examine the extremities for diminished or absent peripheral pulses, edema, and bilateral inequality of pulses; and perform a neurological examination to check for signs of cerebral thrombosis or hemorrhage.

Test-Taking Strategy: Focus on the subject, assessment of a client with hypertension. Recalling that the target organs affected by hypertension are the heart and blood vessels, eyes, brain, and kidneys will assist in answering correctly. Review assessment of a client with hypertension if you had difficulty with this question.

Level of Cognitive Ability: Analysis
Client Needs: Physiological Integrity
Integrated Process: Nursing Process/Assessment
Content Area: Physiological Adaptation

Reference
Black J, Hawks J: *Medical-surgical nursing: clinical management for positive outcomes,* ed 7, Philadelphia, 2005, Saunders, p 1496.

Multiple Response

200. The nurse is preparing a teaching plan about lifestyle modifications for lowering blood pressure. Which of the following should the nurse include in the teaching plan? Select all that apply.

- ❑ 1 Weight reduction
- ❑ 2 Sodium restriction
- ❑ 3 Relaxation techniques
- ❑ 4 Limitation of smoking
- ❑ 5 Restriction of alcohol intake
- ❑ 6 Regular program of exercise

Answer: 1, 2, 3, 5, 6

Rationale: Lifestyle modifications are effective in lowering blood pressure and reducing cardiovascular risk factors. For many people with hypertension whose body weight is more than 10% greater than ideal, weight reduction of as little as 10 pounds can lower blood pressure. Nicotine increases the heart rate and produces peripheral vasoconstriction, which raises arterial blood pressure; therefore smoking needs to be stopped, not limited. Sodium restriction can lower blood pressure. A variety of relaxation therapies, including transcendental meditation, yoga, biofeedback, progressive muscle relaxation, and psychotherapy, can reduce blood pressure in hypertensive clients, at least transiently. The consumption of more than 1 ounce of alcohol a day can elevate the blood pressure; therefore alcohol intake should be restricted. Blood pressure can also be reduced with a regular exercise program.

Test-Taking Strategy: Focus on the subject, lifestyle modifications for lowering blood pressure. Think about the pathophysiology associated with hypertension to answer the question. Also noting the word *limitation* in option 4 will assist in eliminating this option. Review lifestyle modifications for lowering blood pressure if you had difficulty with this question.

Level of Cognitive Ability: Application
Client Needs: Health Promotion and Maintenance
Integrated Process: Teaching and Learning
Content Area: Prevention and Detection of Health Alterations

Reference
Black J, Hawks J: *Medical-surgical nursing: clinical management for positive outcomes,* ed 7, Philadelphia, 2005, Saunders, pp 1498-1499.

Multiple Response

201. Identify the measures that promote venous return in a client with venous stasis. Select all that apply.

- ❑ **1** Bed rest
- ❑ **2** Ambulation
- ❑ **3** Compression stockings
- ❑ **4** Passive range-of-motion (ROM) exercises
- ❑ **5** Placing the foot of the bed in a dependent position
- ❑ **6** Intermittent sequential compression devices

Answer: 2, 3, 4, 6

Rationale: Venous stasis is a disorder in which the normal flow of blood through a vein is slowed or halted. Venous stasis is improved by any activity that causes the leg muscles to contract. Leg exercises and ambulation promote venous return, as do passive ROM exercises. Other methods of promoting venous return include elevating the foot of the bed, applying compression stockings, and using motorized compressive devices.

Test-Taking Strategy: Focus on the subject, measures that promote venous return. Recall that venous stasis is a disorder in which the normal flow of blood through a vein is slowed or halted. Read each option and visualize its effect on blood flow. This will assist in answering correctly. Review the measures that promote venous return if you had difficulty with this question.

Level of Cognitive Ability: Application
Client Needs: Health Promotion and Maintenance
Integrated Process: Nursing Process/Implementation
Content Area: Prevention and Detection of Health Alterations

References
Black J, Hawks J: Medical-surgical nursing: clinical management for positive outcomes, ed 7, Philadelphia, 2005, Saunders, p 1536.
Mosby's medical, nursing, and allied health dictionary, ed 7, St Louis, 2006, Mosby, p 1949.

Multiple Response

202. The nurse provides a pregnant client with which information about relieving nausea and vomiting? Select all that apply.

- ❑ **1** Avoid spicy foods.
- ❑ **2** Eat 5 or 6 small meals a day.
- ❑ **3** Eat a protein snack at bedtime.
- ❑ **4** Drink fluids separately from meals.
- ❑ **5** Eat dry crackers or toast before arising in the morning.
- ❑ **6** Eat small amounts of fatty foods frequently during the day.

Answer: 1, 2, 3, 4, 5

Rationale: Nausea and vomiting of pregnancy are frequently called morning sickness because they are more acute on arising. However, nausea and vomiting can occur at any time of the day. Some measures to relieve this discomfort include eating dry crackers or toast before arising in the morning, then getting out of bed slowly; eating small amounts of carbohydrate foods frequently during the day and 5 or 6 small meals a day; drinking fluids separately from meals; avoiding fatty and spicy foods and those with strong odors; and eating a protein snack at bedtime.

Test-Taking Strategy: Focus on the subject, measures to relieve nausea and vomiting. Read each option, thinking about how it may relieve or prevent nausea. This will assist in selecting the correct options. Also noting the word *fatty* in option 6 will assist in eliminating this option. Review the measures to relieve nausea and vomiting if you had difficulty with this question.

Level of Cognitive Ability: Application
Client Needs: Health Promotion and Maintenance
Integrated Process: Nursing Process/Implementation
Content Area: Growth and Transitions Across the Life Span

Reference
McKinney E, James S, Murray S, et al: *Maternal-child nursing*, ed 2, Philadelphia, 2005, Saunders, p 1210.

Multiple Response

203. A nurse is caring for a pregnant client who is at 32 weeks of gestation with mild preeclampsia. The nurse should be alert to which manifestations that indicate worsening of the condition? Select all that apply.

- ❑ **1** Visual problems
- ❑ **2** Severe headache
- ❑ **3** Decreased platelets
- ❑ **4** Elevated blood glucose
- ❑ **5** Elevated serum creatinine
- ❑ **6** Lower abdominal discomfort

Answer: 1, 2, 3, 5

Rationale: Preeclampsia is a pregnancy-specific syndrome in which hypertension develops after 20 weeks of gestation in a previously normotensive woman. It is characterized by the presence of hypertension and proteinuria. Preeclampsia is usually categorized as mild or severe in terms of management. Visual problems, severe headache, thrombocytopenia (decreased platelets), epigastric pain (from the distention of the liver capsule), and elevated serum creatinine (altered renal function) are manifestations of severe preeclampsia. Elevated blood glucose is found in diabetes mellitus, which is a risk factor associated with the development of preeclampsia.

Test-Taking Strategy: Focus on the subject, manifestations of worsening preeclampsia. Think about the pathophysiology of severe preeclampsia. Option 4 can be eliminated because it relates to diabetes mellitus, not preeclampsia. Recalling that epigastric pain (not lower abdominal discomfort) occurs will assist in eliminating option 6. Review the manifestations of worsening preeclampsia if you had difficulty with this question.

Level of Cognitive Ability: Analysis
Client Needs: Physiological Integrity
Integrated Process: Nursing Process/Assessment
Content Area: Physiological Adaptation

Reference
Wong D, Perry S, Hockenberry M, et al: *Maternal child nursing care*, ed 3, St Louis, 2006, Mosby, p 372

Multiple Response

204. What clinical manifestations would the nurse expect to find in a client who has deep venous thrombosis (DVT)? Select all that apply.

❏ 1 Dilated veins
❏ 2 Low-grade fever
❏ 3 Bilateral leg swelling
❏ 4 Pain in the affected extremity
❏ 5 Pale-colored affected extremity
❏ 6 Coolness of the affected extremity

Answer: 1, 2, 4

Rationale: DVT is a disorder involving a thrombus in one of the deep veins of the body, most commonly the iliac or femoral vein. The clinical manifestations include unilateral leg swelling; pain and redness or warmth of the leg; dilated veins; and a low-grade fever.

Test-Taking Strategy: Focus on the subject, DVT, and think about the pathophysiology of this disorder. This will assist in eliminating option 3 because of the word *bilateral,* option 5 because of the word *pale,* and option 6 because of the word *coolness.* Review the manifestations of DVT if you had difficulty with this question.

Level of Cognitive Ability: Analysis
Client Needs: Physiological Integrity
Integrated Process: Nursing Process/Assessment
Content Area: Physiological Adaptation

Reference
Black J, Hawks J: *Medical-surgical nursing: clinical management for positive outcomes,* ed 7, Philadelphia, 2005, Saunders, p 1537.

Multiple Response

205. The nurse takes which actions to treat a client who develops an anterior nosebleed? Select all that apply.

- ❏ **1** Reassure the client.
- ❏ **2** Keep the client quiet.
- ❏ **3** Apply ice or cool compresses to the nose and face.
- ❏ **4** Assist the client to a right side–lying supine position.
- ❏ **5** Apply direct lateral pressure to the nose for 5 minutes.
- ❏ **6** Instruct the client not to blow the nose for several hours after the bleeding stops.

Answer: 1, 2, 3, 5, 6

Rationale: Immediate care for a client who develops a nosebleed includes positioning the client upright and leaning forward to prevent blood from entering the stomach and possible aspiration; reassuring the client and attempting to keep the client quiet to reduce anxiety and blood pressure; applying direct lateral pressure to the nose for 5 minutes; applying ice or cool compresses to the nose and face if possible; and loosely packing both nares with gauze or nasal tampons if necessary. The client is instructed not to blow the nose for several hours after the bleeding stops to prevent rebleeding from dislodging clots and to seek medical assistance if the rebleeding occurs.

Test-Taking Strategy: Recall that the goals of care are to stop the bleeding, prevent blood from entering the stomach and possible aspiration, and prevent its recurrence. Read each option, keeping these goals in mind. Also note that the only incorrect option contains the word *supine*. The supine position could result in blood entering the stomach and possible aspiration. Review interventions for a nosebleed if you had difficulty with this question.

Level of Cognitive Ability: Application
Client Needs: Physiological Integrity
Integrated Process: Nursing Process/Implementation
Content Area: Physiological Adaptation

Reference
Ignatavicius D, Workman M: *Medical surgical nursing: critical thinking for collaborative care,* ed 5, Philadelphia, 2006, Saunders, p 565.

Multiple Response

206. The nurse is performing an admission assessment on a client who has been diagnosed with a cardiovascular disease. The nurse expects to note which subjective and objective findings? Select all that apply.

❏ 1 Fatigue
❏ 2 Chest pain
❏ 3 Weight loss
❏ 4 Lightheadedness
❏ 5 Dependent edema
❏ 6 Difficulty breathing in an upright position

Answer: 1, 2, 4, 5

Rationale: Cardiovascular disease is any abnormal condition characterized by dysfunction of the heart and blood vessels. Common clinical manifestations of cardiovascular disease include chest pain, irregularities of the heart rhythm, cyanosis, fatigue, lightheadedness, weight gain, dependent edema, and respiratory manifestations such as dyspnea. The client complains of difficulty breathing when lying in a flat position.

Test-Taking Strategy: Focus on the subject, cardiovascular disease. Recall that cardiovascular disease is characterized by dysfunction of the heart and blood vessels, and think about the manifestations of this dysfunction. This will direct you to the correct options. Also note the word *loss* in option 3 and the words *upright position* in option 6. Review the manifestations of cardiovascular disease if you had difficulty with this question.

Level of Cognitive Ability: Analysis
Client Needs: Physiological Integrity
Integrated Process: Nursing Process/Assessment
Content Area: Physiological Adaptation

Reference
Black J, Hawks J: *Medical-surgical nursing: clinical management for positive outcomes,* ed 7, Philadelphia, 2005, Saunders, p 1562.

Multiple Response

207. A nurse is performing an assessment of a client diagnosed with aortic stenosis. What clinical manifestations would the nurse expect the client to exhibit? Select all that apply.

- ❑ **1** Chest pain
- ❑ **2** Syncope at rest
- ❑ **3** Exertional dyspnea
- ❑ **4** Water hammer pulse
- ❑ **5** Pulsations in the neck
- ❑ **6** Paroxysmal nocturnal dyspnea

Answer: 1, 2, 3, 6

Rationale: Aortic stenosis is a narrowing or stricture of the aortic valve. Manifestations begin to appear as the obstruction and ventricular pressure increase to critical levels. Angina pectoris (chest pain) is a frequent finding. Syncope also occurs during exertion because of a fixed cardiac output during a period of increased demand. Syncope at rest may be due to dysrhythmias. Exertional dyspnea and paroxysmal nocturnal dyspnea also occur. In severe aortic stenosis, additional manifestations may include palpitations, fatigue, and visual disturbances. A systolic thrill is present over the aortic areas. A water hammer pulse (Corrigan's pulse) is a bounding pulse in which a great surge is felt, followed by a sudden and complete absence of force or fullness in the artery. A water hammer pulse is associated with aortic regurgitation. Pulsations in the neck are characteristic of tricuspid stenosis or aortic regurgitation.

Test-Taking Strategy: Focus on the subject, aortic stenosis. Think about the action and function of the aortic valve and the pathophysiology associated with stenosis to assist in answering this question. Remember that pulsations in the neck are characteristic of tricuspid stenosis or aortic regurgitation, and a water hammer pulse is associated with aortic regurgitation. Review the manifestations of aortic stenosis if you had difficulty with this question.

Level of Cognitive Ability: Analysis
Client Needs: Physiological Integrity
Integrated Process: Nursing Process/Assessment
Content Area: Physiological Adaptation

Reference
Black J, Hawks J: *Medical-surgical nursing: clinical management for positive outcomes*, ed 7, Philadelphia, 2005, Saunders, p 1603.

Multiple Response

208. A nurse is monitoring a client closely for manifestations of cardiac tamponade. Which of the following are manifestations of this life-threatening condition? Select all that apply.

- ❑ 1 Bradycardia
- ❑ 2 Hypertension
- ❑ 3 Kussmaul's sign
- ❑ 4 Muffled heart sounds
- ❑ 5 Widened pulse pressure
- ❑ 6 Distended neck veins on inspiration

Answer: 3, 4, 6

Rationale: Cardiac tamponade is a life-threatening condition caused by the accumulation of fluid in the pericardium. This fluid, which can be blood, pus, or air in the pericardial sac, accumulates fast and in sufficient quantity to compress the heart and restrict blood flow in and out of the ventricles. The following are manifestations of cardiac tamponade and should be reported immediately: elevated venous pressure, distended neck veins, and Kussmaul's sign (distended neck veins on inspiration); hypotension and narrowed pulse pressure; tachycardia; dyspnea, restlessness, and anxiety; cyanosis of the lips and nails; diaphoresis; muffled heart sounds; pulsus paradoxus; decreased friction rub; decreased QRS voltage; and electrical alternans.

Test-Taking Strategy: Focus on the subject, manifestations of cardiac tamponade. To answer correctly, think about how each option relates to the pathophysiology of this condition. Review the manifestations of cardiac tamponade if you had difficulty with this question.

Level of Cognitive Ability: Analysis
Client Needs: Physiological Integrity
Integrated Process: Nursing Process/Assessment
Content Area: Physiological Adaptation

Reference
Black J, Hawks J: *Medical-surgical nursing: clinical management for positive outcomes,* ed 7, Philadelphia, 2005, Saunders, p 1623.

Multiple Response

209. In caring for a client with infective endocarditis, the nurse expects to note which of the following manifestations of embolization? Select all that apply.

- ❑ 1 Aphasia
- ❑ 2 Petechiae
- ❑ 3 Loss of vision
- ❑ 4 Janeway's lesions
- ❑ 5 Splinter hemorrhages
- ❑ 6 Negative blood culture

Answer: 1, 2, 3, 4, 5

Rationale: Endocarditis is an inflammatory process of the endocardium, especially the valves. Clinical manifestations of infective endocarditis include those related to the infectious process, embolization, and the immune response. Embolization occurs when a vessel is obstructed by vegetations that develop as a result of the disorder. Clinical manifestations related to embolization can occur in any part of the body and include stroke, transient ischemic attacks, aphasia, or ataxia; loss of vision from embolization to the brain or retinal artery; and petechiae on the neck, conjunctiva, chest, abdomen, and mouth. Other manifestations include Roth's spots, a bright red, irregular halo with a white or yellow center seen by ophthalmoscope; myocardial infarction; pulmonary embolus; splinter hemorrhages, which look like tiny splinters under the nail; Osler's nodes, which are painful, erythematous, pea-sized nodules on the tips of the fingers and toes resulting from inflammation around a small, infected embolus; finger clubbing; and Janeway's lesions, which are flat, small, nontender red spots on the palms of the hands and the soles of the feet. The blood culture would be positive and would identify the offending organism.

Test-Taking Strategy: Think about the pathophysiology of infective endocarditis. The strategic word *infective* will assist in eliminating the only incorrect option, option 6. Review the complications associated with infective endocarditis if you had difficulty with this question.

Level of Cognitive Ability: Analysis
Client Needs: Physiological Integrity
Integrated Process: Nursing Process/Assessment
Content Area: Physiological Adaptation

Reference
Black J, Hawks J: *Medical-surgical nursing: clinical management for positive outcomes,* ed 7, Philadelphia, 2005, Saunders, p 1618.

Multiple Response

210. In caring for a client with infective endocarditis, the nurse should be alert for which of the following clinical manifestations related to the infection? Select all that apply.

- ❏ **1** Backache
- ❏ **2** Petechiae
- ❏ **3** Weight loss
- ❏ **4** Osler's nodes
- ❏ **5** Splenomegaly
- ❏ **6** Chills alternating with sweats

Answer: 1, 3, 5, 6

Rationale: Endocarditis is an inflammatory process of the endocardium, especially the valves. Clinical manifestations of infective endocarditis include those related to the infectious process, embolization, and the immune response. Clinical manifestations related to the infection include fever, chills alternating with sweats, malaise, weakness, anorexia, weight loss, pallor, backache, and splenomegaly. The client may report feeling as though he or she has the flu, with headaches and musculoskeletal aching. Petechiae and Osler's nodes are manifestations of embolization, a complication of infective endocarditis.

Test-Taking Strategy: Think about the pathophysiology and the complications that occur in infective endocarditis and focus on the subject, manifestations related to the infection. Remember that petechiae and Osler's nodes are manifestations of embolization, a complication of infective endocarditis. Review the complications associated with infective endocarditis if you had difficulty with this question.

Level of Cognitive Ability: Analysis
Client Needs: Physiological Integrity
Integrated Process: Nursing Process/Assessment
Content Area: Physiological Adaptation

Reference
Black J, Hawks J: *Medical-surgical nursing: clinical management for positive outcomes,* ed 7, Philadelphia, 2005, Saunders, p 1618

Multiple Response

211. A nurse understands that which of the following are indications for creation of a tracheostomy? Select all that apply.

- ❑ **1** Bilateral vocal cord paralysis
- ❑ **2** Prolonged endotracheal tube insertion
- ❑ **3** Access for continuous mechanical ventilation
- ❑ **4** Relief of acute or chronic upper airway obstruction
- ❑ **5** Chemotherapy administration through an implanted port
- ❑ **6** Parenteral nutrition administration through a central intravenous access device

Answer: 1, 2, 3, 4

Rationale: A tracheotomy is a surgical incision into the trachea through overlying skin and muscles for airway management. A tracheostomy is the surgical creation of a stoma, or opening, into the trachea through the underlying skin. Indications for creation of a tracheostomy include bilateral vocal cord paralysis, prolonged endotracheal tube insertion resulting in erosion or pain, access for continuous mechanical ventilation, relief of acute or chronic upper airway obstruction, prevention of aspiration pneumonia, and promotion of pulmonary hygiene. A tracheostomy bypasses the upper airway and glottis, making stabilization, suction, and the attachment of respiratory equipment much easier than with other types of artificial airways. The client can eat and, with some adjustments, talk. Chemotherapy administration through an implanted port and parenteral nutrition administration through a central intravenous access device are not indications for a tracheostomy.

Test-Taking Strategy: Focus on the subject, indications for creation of a tracheostomy. Recall that a tracheostomy is the surgical creation of a stoma into the trachea through the underlying skin, and use the ABCs, airway, breathing, and circulation, to direct you to the correct options. Review the indications for creation of a tracheostomy if you had difficulty with this question.

Level of Cognitive Ability: Analysis
Client Needs: Physiological Integrity
Integrated Process: Nursing Process/Analysis
Content Area: Physiological Adaptation

Reference
Black J, Hawks J: *Medical-surgical nursing: clinical management for positive outcomes,* ed 7, Philadelphia, 2005, Saunders, p 1775.

Prioritizing (Ordered Response)

212. In order of priority, select the steps the nurse takes if a tracheostomy tube is accidentally dislodged and another needs to be inserted because of the inability to maintain ventilation and oxygenation by resuscitation bag and mask. (Number 1 is the first action and number 6 is the last action.)

___ Call for help.

___ Auscultate for breath sounds.

___ Insert the inner cannula, and reconnect it to oxygen and ventilation equipment.

___ Elevate the person's shoulders with a pillow, and gently hyperextend the neck.

___ Insert the outer cannula with obturator into the client's neck, then immediately remove the obturator.

___ Deflate the cuff on a new tracheostomy tube, remove its inner cannula, and insert the obturator in the outer cannula.

Answer: 1, 5, 6, 3, 4, 2

Rationale: A tracheostomy tube that is not properly secured may be accidentally dislodged from the stoma. Manipulation of a tracheostomy tube or suctioning often produces vigorous coughing, which can expel the tube from the stoma unless the tube is held firmly. If extubation occurs, the nurse calls for help immediately and maintains ventilation and oxygenation by resuscitation bag and mask. If ventilation is impossible, the nurse must reinsert the tube if tracheal retention sutures are not present. The procedure should be done in the following order: (1) deflate the cuff on the new tracheostomy tube, remove its inner cannula, and insert the obturator in the outer cannula; (2) elevate the client's shoulders with a pillow, and gently hyperextend the neck (tracheal dilators or spreaders may be needed to hold the stoma open); (3) insert the outer cannula with the obturator in place into the client's neck, and immediately remove the obturator; (4) auscultate for breath sounds; and (6) if breath sounds are present, insert the inner cannula and reconnect it to oxygen and ventilation equipment. If the tracheostomy tube cannot be reinserted in 1 minute, the nurse should call a code for respiratory arrest.

Test-Taking Strategy: Focus on the subject, the procedure for reinserting a tracheostomy tube. Visualize this procedure and each of the actions in the options to identify the correct order of action. Remember that the nurse immediately calls for help and quickly prepares for reinsertion. Review this procedure if you had difficulty with this question.

Level of Cognitive Ability: Application
Client Needs: Physiological Integrity
Integrated Process: Nursing Process/Implementation
Content Area: Physiological Adaptation

Reference
Black J, Hawks J: *Medical-surgical nursing: clinical management for positive outcomes,* ed 7, Philadelphia, 2005, Saunders, p 1780.

Fill-in-the-Blank

213. A nurse performs a health history on a client with a respiratory disorder who indicates that he is a cigarette smoker and that he has smoked two packs a day for the past 30 years. Based on the client's smoking history, what are the pack years?

Answer: _____ **pack years**

Answer: 60

Rationale: Pack years are the number of packs of cigarettes smoked per day multiplied by the number of smoking years. A client who has smoked two packs a day for the past 30 years has a pack year of 60.

Test-Taking Strategy: This question will be easy to answer correctly if you are familiar with the formula for determining pack years in a client's smoking history. Remember that pack years is the number of packs of cigarettes smoked per day multiplied by the number of smoking years. Once you have calculated the answer, verify it using a calculator. Review respiratory assessment and calculation of pack years in a client who smokes if you had difficulty with this question.

Level of Cognitive Ability: Application
Client Needs: Health Promotion and Maintenance
Integrated Process: Nursing Process/Assessment
Content Area: Prevention and Detection of Health Alterations

Reference
Ignatavicius D, Workman M: *Medical surgical nursing: critical thinking for collaborative care*, ed 5, Philadelphia, 2006, Saunders, p 529.

Figure/Illustration with a Multiple Choice

214. The nurse is performing which physical assessment technique? (Refer to figure.)

❑ 1 Palpation
❑ 2 Inspection
❑ 3 Percussion
❑ 4 Auscultation

Answer: 3

Rationale: Percussion involves striking a finger or hand directly against the client's body. The nurse may use one or both hands to percuss, depending on which body system is being assessed. Inspection involves a visual examination of the body. Palpation involves the use of the nurse's hands to feel texture, size, shape, consistency, and location of certain parts of the body and to identify areas that the client reports as being painful or tender. Auscultation is the act of listening to sounds within the body.

Test-Taking Strategy: Focus on the figure. Recalling the techniques used in physical assessment and their description will assist in answering correctly. Review these physical assessment techniques if you had difficulty with this question.

Level of Cognitive Ability: Analysis
Client Needs: Health Promotion and Maintenance
Integrated Process: Nursing Process/Assessment
Content Area: Prevention and Detection of Health Alterations

References
Ignatavicius D, Workman M: *Medical surgical nursing: critical thinking for collaborative care,* ed 5, Philadelphia, 2006, Saunders, p 533.
Wilson S, Giddens J: *Health assessment for nursing practice,* ed 3, St Louis, 2005, Mosby, pp 55-57.

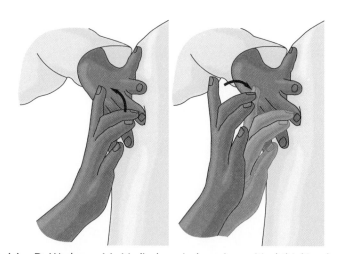

From Ignatavicius D, Workman M: *Medical surgical nursing: critical thinking for collaborative care,* ed 5, Philadelphia, 2006, Saunders.

Multiple Response

215. A nurse is providing home care instructions to a client after a lumbar diskectomy. Which instructions should the nurse provide to the client? Select all that apply.

- ❏ 1 Daily walking is beneficial.
- ❏ 2 Sleeping on a firm mattress is important.
- ❏ 3 Returning to work may be allowed in 4 to 6 weeks.
- ❏ 4 Driving a car is not permitted until allowed by the surgeon.
- ❏ 5 Items can be lifted as long as they weigh less than 10 pounds.
- ❏ 6 Stair climbing is not restricted and can be done as often as necessary.

Answer: 1, 2, 3, 4

Rationale: After a lumbar diskectomy the client is limited in the number of times that he or she can climb stairs. Daily walking is encouraged as a form of exercise. The client should lie on a firm mattress to provide support for the entire vertebral column. The client can usually return to work in 4 to 6 weeks, depending on the job and the extent and type of surgery. Driving is not permitted for several weeks until the client is reevaluated by the surgeon. Items that can be lifted should weigh no more than 5 pounds.

Test-Taking Strategy: Focus on the type of surgery, a lumbar diskectomy. Visualize the location of this surgical procedure, and read each option, thinking about the stress it may place on the surgical area. This will direct you to the correct options. Review home care instructions after having a lumbar diskectomy if you had difficulty with this question.

Level of Cognitive Ability: Application
Client Needs: Physiological Integrity
Integrated Process: Teaching and Learning
Content Area: Reduction of Risk Potential

References

Black J, Hawks J: *Medical-surgical nursing: clinical management for positive outcomes,* ed 7, Philadelphia, 2005, Saunders, p 2149.

Ignatavicius D, Workman M: *Medical surgical nursing: critical thinking for collaborative care,* ed 5, Philadelphia, 2006, Saunders, pp 981-982.

Multiple Response

216. A nurse is caring for a client with dementia. What cognitive activities can the nurse expect to be impaired in the client? Select all that apply.

❏ **1** Memory
❏ **2** Judgment
❏ **3** Bradykinesia
❏ **4** Decision making
❏ **5** Spatial orientation
❏ **6** Verbal communication

Answer: 1, 2, 4, 5, 6

Rationale: The term *dementia* refers to the loss of memory, reasoning, judgment, and language to an extent that it interferes with everyday life. Cognition is the act or process of thinking, perceiving, and learning. Cognitive activities that become impaired in dementia include memory, judgment, decision making, spatial orientation, thinking, reasoning, and verbal communication. A client with dementia may undergo behavioral and personality changes as well, depending on the areas of the brain affected. Bradykinesia is not a cognitive activity, and is a manifestation of Parkinson's disease, not dementia.

Test-Taking Strategy: Focus on the client's diagnosis and the subject of the question, cognitive activities that become impaired. Read each option and determine its relation to the description of dementia and impaired cognition. This will assist in determining the correct options. Review expected findings in the client with dementia if you had difficulty with this question.

Level of Cognitive Ability: Analysis
Client Needs: Physiological Integrity
Integrated Process: Nursing Process/Assessment
Content Area: Physiological Adaptation

Reference

Black J, Hawks J: *Medical-surgical nursing: clinical management for positive outcomes*, ed 7, Philadelphia, 2005, Saunders, pp 2161, 2173.

Multiple Response

217. Which of the following findings would the nurse expect to observe in a client with multi-infarct (multiple stroke) dementia? Select all that apply.

- ❏ **1** Wandering
- ❏ **2** Muscle stiffness
- ❏ **3** Problems managing money
- ❏ **4** Problems with recent memory
- ❏ **5** Difficulty following instructions
- ❏ **6** Laughing or crying inappropriately

Answer: 1, 3, 4, 5, 6

Rationale: Multi-infarct (multiple stroke) disease is a cause of irreversible dementia. Blood clots block small blood vessels in the brain and destroy brain tissue. Manifestations of multi-infarct dementia often develop in a stepwise manner and include problems with recent memory, wandering or getting lost in familiar places, incontinence, emotional lability such as laughing or crying inappropriately, difficulty following instructions, and problems managing money. Muscle stiffness is not a manifestation of this type of dementia, although it can occur in Lewy body dementia, which is similar to Alzheimer's disease.

Test-Taking Strategy: Focus on the client's diagnosis. Noting the strategic words *stroke* and *dementia* will assist in determining the correct options. Also note that the incorrect option is the only option that is a physiological manifestation. The correct options address psychosocial manifestations. Review the manifestations of multi-infarct dementia if you had difficulty with this question.

Level of Cognitive Ability: Analysis
Client Needs: Physiological Integrity
Integrated Process: Nursing Process/Assessment
Content Area: Physiological Adaptation

Reference
Black J, Hawks J: *Medical-surgical nursing: clinical management for positive outcomes,* ed 7, Philadelphia, 2005, Saunders, pp 2164-2165, 2175.

Multiple Response

218. What nonverbal client behaviors can provide clues to the nurse about the specific needs of a distressed client with Alzheimer's disease? Select all that apply.

❑ **1** Hand gesturing
❑ **2** Rattling doorknobs
❑ **3** Decreased motor activity
❑ **4** Tightening facial muscles
❑ **5** Quiet and subdued manner
❑ **6** Waving arms or shaking fists

Answer: 1, 2, 4, 6

Rationale: Alzheimer's disease is a form of dementia. Nonverbal behavior can provide clues about specific needs of a distressed client. Clients with Alzheimer's disease often avert their eyes, look down, back away, and increase hand gesturing when they do not understand. If they are frustrated, angry, or hostile, they may increase motor activity by pacing, rattling doorknobs, waving their arms or shaking their fists, frowning, raising their voice volume and pitch, or tightening their facial muscles. A quiet and subdued manner and decreased motor activity do not indicate distress.

Test-Taking Strategy: Note the strategic words *distressed client*. The only manifestations that do not indicate distress are a quiet and subdued manner and decreased motor activity. Review the nonverbal behaviors that can provide clues about specific needs of a distressed client if you had difficulty with this question.

Level of Cognitive Ability: Analysis
Client Needs: Physiological Integrity
Integrated Process: Nursing Process/Assessment
Content Area: Physiological Adaptation

Reference
Black J, Hawks J: *Medical-surgical nursing: clinical management for positive outcomes,* ed 7, Philadelphia, 2005, Saunders, pp 2167-2168.

Multiple Response

219. A nurse is developing a care plan for a client with Alzheimer's disease who has impaired receptive and expressive language abilities. Which of the following interventions should be part of the care plan? Select all that apply.

❑ 1 Increase environmental stimuli.
❑ 2 Approach the client with assurance.
❑ 3 Encourage verbalization of feelings.
❑ 4 Avoid placing demands on the client.
❑ 5 Use verbal and nonverbal communication cues.
❑ 6 Use multiple sensory modalities one at a time to send the message.

Answer: 2, 4, 5, 6

Rationale: Alzheimer's disease is a form of dementia. When the client's receptive and expressive language abilities are impaired, the nurse must be prepared to adapt to the communication level of the client. Interventions can include decreasing environmental stimuli; approaching the client calmly and with assurance; taking care not to place any demands on the client; gently distracting the client; ensuring that all verbal and nonverbal communication cues are concordant; and using multiple sensory modalities (visual, auditory, and tactile) to send the message (though not all modalities should be used at the same time).

Test-Taking Strategy: Focus on the client's diagnosis and the subject of the question, impaired receptive and expressive language abilities. This will assist in determining that options 1 and 3 are incorrect. Review interventions for the client with impaired receptive and expressive language abilities if you had difficulty with this question.

Level of Cognitive Ability: Application
Client Needs: Psychosocial Integrity
Integrated Process: Nursing Process/Planning
Content Area: Mental Health Disorders

Reference
Black J, Hawks J: *Medical-surgical nursing: clinical management for positive outcomes,* ed 7, Philadelphia, 2005, Saunders, pp 2167-2168.

Multiple Response

220. The nurse is performing an assessment of a client who has Parkinson's disease (PD). The nurse expects to note which primary manifestations of this disorder? Select all that apply.

- ❏ **1** Rigidity
- ❏ **2** Bradykinesia
- ❏ **3** Tremor at rest
- ❏ **4** Intellectual decline
- ❏ **5** Loss of postural reflexes
- ❏ **6** Flexed posture of the neck

Answer: 1, 2, 3, 5, 6

Rationale: PD is a chronic, progressive, neurological disorder that results from the loss of the neurotransmitter dopamine in a group of brain structures that control movements. The disease has six primary manifestations: (1) tremor at rest; (2) rigidity; (3) bradykinesia (slow movement); (4) flexed posture of the neck, trunk, and limbs; (5) loss of postural reflexes; and (6) freezing movement. Intellectual decline is not a manifestation; usually PD does not affect intellectual ability.

Test-Taking Strategy: Focus on the client's diagnosis. Recalling that PD results from the loss of the neurotransmitter dopamine, which controls movements, will assist in determining the correct manifestations. Review these primary manifestations if you had difficulty with this question.

Level of Cognitive Ability: Analysis
Client Needs: Physiological Integrity
Integrated Process: Nursing Process/Assessment
Content Area: Physiological Adaptation

Reference
Black J, Hawks J: *Medical-surgical nursing: clinical management for positive outcomes,* ed 7, Philadelphia, 2005, Saunders, pp 2170-2172.

Multiple Response

221. In caring for a client with myasthenia gravis, the nurse should be alert for which of the following manifestations of cholinergic crisis? Select all that apply.

❑ **1** Blurred vision
❑ **2** Fasciculations
❑ **3** Abdominal cramps
❑ **4** Increased heart rate
❑ **5** Decreased secretions and saliva
❑ **6** Weakness with difficulty swallowing

Answer: 1, 2, 3, 6

Rationale: Clients with myasthenia gravis may experience a cholinergic crisis as a result of overmedication. Clinical manifestations include weakness with difficulty swallowing, chewing, speaking, and breathing; apprehension; nausea and vomiting; abdominal cramps and diarrhea; increased secretions and saliva; sweating; lacrimation; fasciculations; and blurred vision. Increased heart rate is not associated with cholinergic crisis, although it may be a manifestation of myasthenic crisis.

Test-Taking Strategy: Recall that clients with myasthenia gravis are treated with anticholinesterase medications and that cholinergic crisis occurs as a result of overmedication. Think about the adverse effects of overmedication with an anticholinesterase to select the correct options. Review the manifestations of cholinergic crisis if you had difficulty with this question.

Level of Cognitive Ability: Analysis
Client Needs: Physiological Integrity
Integrated Process: Nursing Process/Assessment
Content Area: Physiological Adaptation

Reference

Black J, Hawks J: *Medical-surgical nursing: clinical management for positive outcomes,* ed 7, Philadelphia, 2005, Saunders, p 2184.

Multiple Response

222. A nurse is caring for a client who has degeneration of the lower motor neurons related to amyotrophic lateral sclerosis. What clinical manifestations would the nurse expect to note during assessment of the client? Select all that apply.

- ❏ **1** Atrophy
- ❏ **2** Cramps
- ❏ **3** Spasticity
- ❏ **4** Weakness
- ❏ **5** Hyperreflexia
- ❏ **6** Fasciculations

Answer: 1, 2, 4, 6

Rationale: Amyotrophic lateral sclerosis involves degeneration of both the anterior horn cells and the corticospinal tracts. Consequently, both upper and lower motor neuron clinical manifestations are seen. Lower motor neuron clinical manifestations include weakness, atrophy, cramps, and fasciculations (irregular twitching of muscle fibers or bundles). Upper motor neuron manifestations include spasticity and hyperreflexia.

Test-Taking Strategy: Note the strategic words *lower motor neurons*. Specific knowledge regarding the manifestations associated with both upper and lower motor neuron degeneration is needed to answer correctly. However, if you can remember that upper motor neuron manifestations include spasticity and hyperreflexia, you will be able to answer questions similar to this one. Review the manifestations of both upper and lower motor neuron degeneration if you had difficulty with this question.

Level of Cognitive Ability: Analysis
Client Needs: Physiological Integrity
Integrated Process: Nursing Process/Assessment
Content Area: Physiological Adaptation

Reference

Black J, Hawks J: *Medical-surgical nursing: clinical management for positive outcomes,* ed 7, Philadelphia, 2005, Saunders, p 2185.

Multiple Response

223. A nurse is monitoring a male client with a spinal cord injury who is experiencing spinal shock. The nurse monitors for which indications that the spinal shock is resolving? Select all that apply.

- ❏ 1 Flaccidity
- ❏ 2 Presence of a gag reflex
- ❏ 3 Positive Babinski's reflex
- ❏ 4 Development of hyperreflexia
- ❏ 5 Return of the bulbocavernous reflex
- ❏ 6 Return of reflex emptying of the bladder

Answer: 3, 4, 5, 6

Rationale: Spinal shock is associated with acute injury to the spinal cord with temporary suppression of reflexes controlled by segments below the level of injury. It may last for 1 to 6 weeks. Indications that spinal shock is resolving include return of reflexes, development of hyperreflexia rather than flaccidity, and return of reflex emptying of the bladder. The return of the bulbocavernous reflex in male patients is also an early indictor of recovery from spinal shock. Babinski's reflex (dorsiflexion of the great toe with fanning of the other toes when the sole of the foot is stroked) is an early returning reflex. The gag reflex is not lost in spinal shock; therefore its presence is not an indication of resolving spinal shock.

Test-Taking Strategy: Note the strategic words *spinal shock is resolving*. As you read each option, recall that spinal shock is associated with acute injury to the spinal cord with temporary suppression of reflexes controlled by segments below the level of injury. This will assist in eliminating flaccidity and the presence of a gag reflex as signs that spinal shock is resolving. Review the indications that spinal shock is resolving if you had difficulty with this question.

Level of Cognitive Ability: Analysis
Client Needs: Physiological Integrity
Integrated Process: Nursing Process/Evaluation
Content Area: Physiological Adaptation

Reference
Black J, Hawks J: *Medical-surgical nursing: clinical management for positive outcomes,* ed 7, Philadelphia, 2005, Saunders, p 2216.

Multiple Response

224. A nurse is developing a care plan for a client with total urinary incontinence related to paralysis. Appropriate nursing interventions include which of the following? Select all that apply.

❑ 1 Allow bladder distention before catheterization.
❑ 2 Institute measures to prevent urinary tract infections.
❑ 3 Establish and maintain a routine pattern of elimination.
❑ 4 Institute measures to preserve existing bladder capacity.
❑ 5 Institute measures to preserve existing bladder muscle tone.
❑ 6 Institute maximum artificial assistance, such as catheterization, to empty the bladder.

Answer: 2, 3, 4, 5

Rationale: Nursing interventions for a client with total urinary incontinence related to paralysis are planned to prevent urinary tract infections, to preserve existing bladder capacity and muscle tone, and to establish and maintain a routine pattern of elimination requiring minimum artificial assistance. Bladder distention is avoided because it causes stretching and fissure formation, a predisposing factor for bladder infection, and may result in bladder rupture.

Test-Taking Strategy: Focus on the subject, nursing interventions for a client with total urinary incontinence related to paralysis. Eliminate option 1 because allowing bladder distention can result in infection, and eliminate option 6 because of the word *maximum*. Review these nursing interventions if you had difficulty with this question.

Level of Cognitive Ability: Application
Client Needs: Physiological Integrity
Integrated Process: Nursing Process/Planning
Content Area: Basic Care and Comfort

Reference
Black J, Hawks J: *Medical-surgical nursing: clinical management for positive outcomes,* ed 7, Philadelphia, 2005, Saunders, p 2227.

Figure/Illustration with a Fill-in-the-Blank

225. The nurse assesses the volume of lochia based on the amount of staining on the postpartum client's perineal pad. Which finding indicates a moderate amount of lochia flow? (Refer to figure.)

Answer: _____

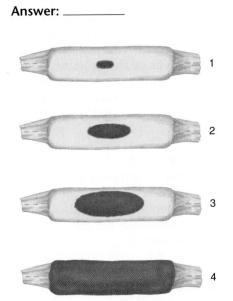

From McKinney E, James S, Murray S, et al: *Maternal-child nursing,* ed 2, Philadelphia, 2005, Saunders.

Answer: 3

Rationale: Lochia flow can be described as either scant (less than a 2.5-cm [1-inch] stain on the perineal pad), light (2.5- to 10-cm [1- to 4-inch] stain), moderate (10- to 15-cm [4- to 6-inch] stain), large (saturated perineal pad in 1 hour), or excessive (saturated perineal pad in 15 minutes).

Test-Taking Strategy: Note the strategic word *moderate.* Recalling that a moderate flow indicates a stain of 4 to 6 inches will assist in directing you to option 3. Review postpartum assessment related to lochia flow if you had difficulty with this question.

Level of Cognitive Ability: Analysis
Client Needs: Health Promotion and Maintenance
Integrated Process: Nursing Process/Assessment
Content Area: Prevention and Detection of Health Alterations

Reference
McKinney E, James S, Murray S, et al: *Maternal-child nursing,* ed 2, Philadelphia, 2005, Saunders, p 467.

Multiple Response

226. Wrist restraints are prescribed for a child after repair of a cleft lip. Select the interventions that the nurse plans during use of the restraints. Select all that apply.

❑ **1** Ensure proper fit of the restraint.
❑ **2** Tie knots that can be easily untied for quick access.
❑ **3** Check the physician's order regarding use of the restraint.
❑ **4** Secure the ties to the mattress or side rails for quick access.
❑ **5** Tell the mother that the restraints must be left on and tied at all times.
❑ **6** Check both wrists for signs of circulatory, integumentary, and neurological compromise before applying the restraint.

Answer: 1, 2, 3, 6

Rationale: To prevent trauma to a surgical site, restraints may be temporarily prescribed. The nurse should always check the physician's order for use of the restraint and ensure that the order states why the restraint is needed and how long it will be in place. The nurse always follows agency policies and procedures regarding the use of restraints. Other interventions include using the least restrictive restraint; choosing the proper restraint for the child's condition; assessing both wrists for signs of circulatory, integumentary, or neurological compromise before applying the restraints and frequently once they are applied; ensuring proper fit of the restraint; tying knots that can be easily untied for quick access; and securing ties to bed frames (not mattresses or side rails). The restraints can be removed while the mother visits as long as the mother remains with the child.

Test-Taking Strategy: Visualize each of the options, keeping safety in mind. This will assist in eliminating option 4 because restraints should be secured to bed frames (not mattresses or side rails). Next eliminate option 5 because of the closed-ended word *must*. Review interventions for the use of restraints if you had difficulty with this question.

Level of Cognitive Ability: Application
Client Needs: Safe and Effective Care Environment
Integrated Process: Nursing Process/Implementation
Content Area: Safety and Infection Control

Reference

McKinney E, James S, Murray S, et al: *Maternal-child nursing,* ed 2, Philadelphia, 2005, Saunders, pp 935-936.

Multiple Response

227. A nurse is teaching a postpartum woman how to bathe her newborn. The nurse provides which instructions to the mother? Select all that apply.

- ❏ **1** Support the newborn's body at all times.
- ❏ **2** Clean any eye discharge using a wet cotton ball.
- ❏ **3** Fill the bathtub with no more than 10 inches of water.
- ❏ **4** Clean the eyes moving from the outer canthus to the inner canthus.
- ❏ **5** Cover the newborn's body except for the part being washed or rinsed.
- ❏ **6** Begin the bath with the face, and clean the newborn's diaper area next.

Answer: 1, 2, 5

Rationale: During bathing, the newborn's body is supported at all times by placing a hand under the newborn's head and neck. If the newborn is bathed in a bathtub, the tub should be lined with a towel to provide comfort and traction to prevent slipping, and it is filled with no more than 3 inches of water. The newborn's body is covered except for the part being washed or rinsed. Any eye discharge is cleaned using a wet cotton ball moving from the inner canthus to the outer canthus. The bath is started with the face, then other body areas are washed, and the diaper area is cleaned last.

Test-Taking Strategy: Visualize each option carefully, keeping the principles of safety and infection control in mind. Eliminate option 3 because of the words *10 inches*. Eliminate option 4 because of the words *outer canthus to the inner canthus*. Eliminate option 6, recalling that the diaper area is cleaned last. Review the procedure for bathing a newborn if you had difficulty with this question.

Level of Cognitive Ability: Application
Client Needs: Health Promotion and Maintenance
Integrated Process: Teaching and Learning
Content Area: Growth and Transitions Across the Life Span

Reference
McKinney E, James S, Murray S, et al: *Maternal-child nursing,* ed 2, Philadelphia, 2005, Saunders, pp 935-936.

Multiple Response

228. The nurse prepares to measure vital signs on an 18-month-old child. The nurse uses which principles as a guide for taking the vital signs? Select all that apply.

- ❏ **1** Count the apical heart rate before taking other vital signs.
- ❏ **2** Count the respirations after taking the child's temperature.
- ❏ **3** Measure the apical heart rate for 30 seconds and multiply the finding by two.
- ❏ **4** Observe the child's respiratory rate and effort for 1 full minute while the child is quiet.
- ❏ **5** Use a tympanic thermometer to measure the temperature if the child has diarrhea.
- ❏ **6** Use a manual cuff to verify electronically measured blood pressures that indicate hypertension or hypotension.

Answer: 1, 4, 5, 6

Rationale: Both respirations and the apical heart rate are counted before taking other vital signs, and both of these signs are measured on a sleeping child or while the child is quiet. The apical heart rate is measured for 1 full minute on any child younger than 2 years. Respirations are also counted for 1 full minute. Temperatures should not be measured rectally in an immunocompromised child or in a child who has had rectal surgery, diarrhea, or a bleeding disorder; tympanic or axillary methods are used instead. A manual cuff should be used to verify electronically measured blood pressures that indicate hypertension or hypotension.

Test-Taking Strategy: Visualize each option and think about the principles for measuring vital signs in a child. Remember that respirations should be measured before other vital signs are taken and that the apical heart rate is counted for 1 full minute. Review these principles if you had difficulty with this question.

Level of Cognitive Ability: Application
Client Needs: Physiological Integrity
Integrated Process: Nursing Process/Assessment
Content Area: Physiological Adaptation

Reference

McKinney E, James S, Murray S, et al: *Maternal-child nursing,* ed 2, Philadelphia, 2005, Saunders, p 940.

Fill-in-the-Blank

229. The nurse is preparing to administer an intramuscular injection into the vastus lateralis muscle of a 3-year-old child. The nurse understands that the maximum safe volume for administration into this site is how many milliliters?

Answer: _____ mL

Answer: 1.5

Rationale: The vastus lateralis is located on the anterior lateral thigh and is well developed at birth. It is a muscle that is able to tolerate large volumes of medication and is not located near vital structures such as nerves or blood vessels. In a young child (3 to 6 years), the maximum safe volume for intramuscular injection into the vastus lateralis muscle is 1.5 mL.

Test-Taking Strategy: Specific knowledge regarding the maximum safe volume for an intramuscular injection into the vastus lateralis muscle is needed to answer this question. Note the strategic words *vastus lateralis* and recall that this is a muscle that is able to tolerate large volumes of medication. Review procedures for administering intramuscular injections to a child if you had difficulty with this question.

Level of Cognitive Ability: Application
Client Needs: Physiological Integrity
Integrated Process: Nursing Process/Implementation
Content Area: Pharmacological and Parenteral Therapies

Reference
McKinney E, James S, Murray S, et al: *Maternal-child nursing,* ed 2, Philadelphia, 2005, Saunders, p 978.

Figure/Illustration with a Fill-in-the-Blank

230. When reviewing the function of the immune system, the nurse understands that which organ or tissue acts as a filter to remove debris and antigens and to foster contact with T lymphocytes? (Refer to figure.)

Answer: _____

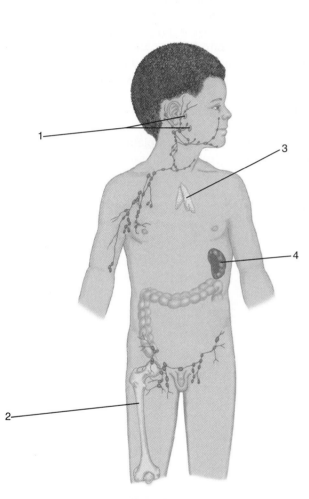

**Major Ogans and Tissues
of the Immune System**

From McKinney E, James S, Murray S, et al: *Maternal-child nursing,* ed 2, Philadelphia, 2005, Saunders.

Answer: 4

Rationale: The spleen acts as a filter to remove debris and antigens and to foster contact with T lymphocytes. Although the tonsils and adenoids (option 1) act as a filter to remove debris and antigens entering the respiratory system, they do not foster contact with T lymphocytes. The bone marrow (option 2) contains stem cells for B lymphocytes, which mature and become antibody-producing plasma cells that react to many bacteria, viruses, and other antigens. The thymus (option 3) contains cells that mature into T lymphocytes and specifically react to viruses, parasites, fungi, foreign tissue, and other antigens. The thymus also controls cell-mediated immunity.

Test-Taking Strategy: Focus on the subject, the organ or tissue that acts as a filter to remove debris and antigens and to foster contact with T lymphocytes. Use knowledge of anatomy and physiology to answer correctly. Review the functions of the organs and tissues of the immune system if you had difficulty with this question.

Level of Cognitive Ability: Analysis
Client Needs: Physiological Integrity
Integrated Process: Nursing Process/Assessment
Content Area: Physiological Adaptation

Reference
McKinney E, James S, Murray S, et al: *Maternal-child nursing,* ed 2, Philadelphia, 2005, Saunders, p 1046.

Multiple Response

231. A pregnant client who is human immunodeficiency virus (HIV) positive asks the nurse about the ways that HIV can be transmitted. The nurse tells the client that HIV is transmitted by which ways? Select all that apply.

❏ 1 Sneezing
❏ 2 Coughing
❏ 3 Breastfeeding
❏ 4 Unprotected sexual activity
❏ 5 Hugging or holding her newborn
❏ 6 Open wounds if there is blood-to-blood contact

Answer: 3, 4, 6

Rationale: HIV infection is an acquired cell-mediated immuno-deficiency disorder that is present in an infected individual's blood or body fluids and can enter an uninfected individual. HIV can be spread by unprotected sexual activity, by sharing of needles, across the placenta during pregnancy, by breast-feeding, or via open wounds if there is blood-to-blood contact. HIV cannot be spread by sharing eating or drinking utensils; using the same toilet seats, bathtubs, or showers; coughing or sneezing; or hugging, holding, or touching others.

Test-Taking Strategy: Focus on the subject, the methods of transmission of HIV. Recalling that HIV infection is present in an infected individual's blood or body fluids will direct you to the correct options. Review methods of transmission of HIV if you had difficulty with this question.

Level of Cognitive Ability: Application
Client Needs: Safe and Effective Care Environment
Integrated Process: Teaching and Learning
Content Area: Safety and Infection Control

Reference
McKinney E, James S, Murray S, et al: *Maternal-child nursing*, ed 2, Philadelphia, 2005, Saunders, p 1058.

Prioritizing (Ordered Response)

232. The nurse prepares to collect a urine specimen from an infant using a collection device. In order of priority, select the steps that the nurse takes to perform this procedure. (Number 1 is the first step and number 6 is the last step.)

____ Put on gloves.

____ Apply the collection bag.

____ Place a diaper on the child.

____ Place the child in a frog-leg position.

____ Clean the perineal area and dry it thoroughly.

____ Remove the backing from the adhesive surface of the collection bag.

Answer: 1, 5, 6, 4, 2, 3

Rationale: To apply a urine collection device or bag, the nurse washes the hands, puts on gloves, and cleans the perineal area to remove any lotions or ointments to help the bag adhere. Drying the perineal area thoroughly will also help the bag adhere. The nurse removes the backing from the adhesive surface of the collection bag, places the child in a frog-leg position, and applies the collection bag. The nurse then places a diaper on the child, cuts a slit in the diaper, and pulls the end of the empty bag through the slit so that the bag protrudes from the diaper. This step reduces the chance of leaking and allows for observation of urine. The bag is checked every 30 minutes for the collection of urine.

Test-Taking Strategy: Visualize this procedure to assist in answering correctly. Remember that the nurse puts gloves on first and places a diaper on the child last. Review this procedure if you had difficulty with this question.

Level of Cognitive Ability: Application
Client Needs: Physiological Integrity
Integrated Process: Nursing Process/Implementation
Content Area: Physiological Adaptation

Reference
McKinney E, James S, Murray S, et al: *Maternal-child nursing,* ed 2, Philadelphia, 2005, Saunders, p 947.

Multiple Response

233. The nurse is preparing an enteral feeding for administration via a nasogastric tube in an infant. The nurse follows which guidelines for administration of the feeding? Select all that apply.

- ❏ **1** Warm the formula in a microwave.
- ❏ **2** Provide a pacifier to the infant during the feeding.
- ❏ **3** Verify tube placement before beginning the feeding.
- ❏ **4** Discard any formula that has been opened for more than 4 hours.
- ❏ **5** If signs of respiratory distress occur, slow the rate of the feeding.
- ❏ **6** Place an amount of formula for a 4-hour feeding in the feeding bag.

Answer: 2, 3, 4, 6

Rationale: Tube feedings are administered at room temperature and are not warmed because of the risk for burns. The nurse always verifies tube placement before beginning the feeding because of the risk of aspiration if the tube is malpositioned. A pacifier is provided to the infant during the feeding so that the infant can associate sucking with feeding. The nurse places an amount of formula for a 4-hour feeding in the feeding bag and discards any formula that has been opened for more than 4 hours. If signs of respiratory distress, cyanosis, abdominal distention, or vomiting occur, the feeding is stopped and the physician is notified.

Test-Taking Strategy: Visualize each option and think about its effect with regard to maintaining safety during feedings. Eliminate option 1, recalling that warming the formula in a microwave can cause burning. Eliminate option 5 because, if signs of respiratory distress occur, the feeding is stopped, not slowed, and the physician is notified. Review the procedure for administering tube feedings if you had difficulty with this question.

Level of Cognitive Ability: Application
Client Needs: Physiological Integrity
Integrated Process: Nursing Process/Implementation
Content Area: Basic Care and Comfort

Reference
McKinney E, James S, Murray S, et al: *Maternal-child nursing,* ed 2, Philadelphia, 2005, Saunders, p 956.

Multiple Response

234. Which of the following are characteristics of right-sided heart failure? Select all that apply.

❑ **1** Weight gain
❑ **2** Dependent edema
❑ **3** Crackles in the lungs
❑ **4** Enlarged liver and spleen
❑ **5** Frothy pink-tinged sputum
❑ **6** Jugular neck vein distention

Answer: 1, 2, 4, 6

Rationale: Heart failure is a condition that refers to the inadequacy of the heart to pump blood throughout the body. The manifestations of right-sided failure reflect the systemic congestion that occurs. These manifestations include jugular neck vein distention, enlarged liver and spleen, anorexia and nausea, dependent edema, distended abdomen, swollen hands and fingers, polyuria at night, weight gain, and hypertension. The manifestations of left-sided heart failure are respiratory and reflect the pulmonary congestion that occurs. These manifestations include a hacking cough that worsens at night, dyspnea and breathlessness, crackles or wheezes in the lungs, and frothy or pink-tinged sputum.

Test-Taking Strategy: Note the subject of the question, manifestations of right-sided heart failure. Remember that the manifestations of right-sided failure affect the systemic circulation. Also remember *"left and lungs"* to assist in determining the manifestations of left-sided heart failure. Review the manifestations of right-sided and left-sided heart failure if you had difficulty with this question.

Level of Cognitive Ability: Analysis
Client Needs: Physiological Integrity
Integrated Process: Nursing Process/Assessment
Content Area: Physiological Adaptation

Reference

Ignatavicius D, Workman M: *Medical surgical nursing: critical thinking for collaborative care,* ed 5, Philadelphia, 2006, Saunders, p 753.

Multiple Response

235. The nurse is caring for a client with tuberculosis (TB) and assesses for which manifestations of this disease? Select all that apply.

❑ **1** Weight gain
❑ **2** Night sweats
❑ **3** Low-grade fever
❑ **4** Increased appetite
❑ **5** Lethargy and fatigue
❑ **6** Cough with mucopurulent sputum

Answer: 2, 3, 5, 6

Rationale: TB is a highly communicable disease caused by *Mycobacterium tuberculosis* that is transmitted via the airborne route. The client with TB has progressive fatigue, lethargy, nausea, anorexia, weight loss, irregular menses, and a low-grade fever. Night sweats may occur, and the client has a cough with mucopurulent sputum, which may be streaked with blood. Chest tightness and a dull aching chest pain occur with the cough.

Test-Taking Strategy: Focus on the client's diagnosis. Recalling that this disease is a highly communicable one that is transmitted via the airborne route will assist in answering this question. Also, eliminate options 1 and 4 because weight loss and anorexia occur in this disorder. Review the manifestations of TB if you had difficulty with this question.

Level of Cognitive Ability: Application
Client Needs: Physiological Integrity
Integrated Process: Nursing Process/Assessment
Content Area: Physiological Adaptation

Reference

Ignatavicius D, Workman M: *Medical surgical nursing: critical thinking for collaborative care,* ed 5, Philadelphia, 2006, Saunders, p 641.

Fill-in-the-Blank

236. The nurse hangs an intravenous (IV) bag of 1000 mL of normal saline at 1 PM and sets to flow rate to infuse at 125 mL/hr. At 5 PM the nurse would expect that how many milliliters of fluid will remain in the IV bag?

Answer: _____ mL

Answer: 500

Rationale: In an 4-hour period, 500 mL would infuse if an IV is set to infuse at 125 mL/hr. Therefore 500 mL would remain in the IV bag.

Test-Taking Strategy: Focus on the data in the question and use simple math to determine that in a 4-hour period (1 to 5 PM), 500 mL would infuse (4 hr × 125 mL/hr = 500 mL). This means that 500 mL would remain. Perform the calculation, and then verify your answer using a calculator. Review calculations related to IV infusions if you had difficulty with this question.

Level of Cognitive Ability: Comprehension
Client Needs: Physiological Integrity
Integrated Process: Nursing Process/Evaluation
Content Area: Pharmacological and Parenteral Therapies

Reference
Kee J, Marshall S: *Clinical calculations: with applications to general and specialty areas,* ed 5, Philadelphia, 2004, Saunders, p 202.

Figure/Illustration with a Fill-in-the-Blank

237. The physician orders 12 mEq of liquid potassium chloride. The medication label reads 20 mEq/15 mL. The nurse prepares the medication and fills the medication cup to which point to administer the correct amount? (Refer to figure.)

Answer: _____

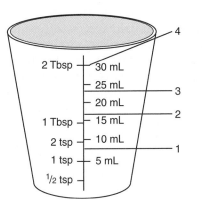

From Macklin D, Chernecky C, Infortuna H: *Math for clinical practice,* St Louis, 2005, Mosby.

Answer: 1

Rationale: Use the formula for calculating medication doses.

Formula

$$\frac{\text{Desired} \times \text{mL}}{\text{Available}} = \text{mL per dose}$$

$$\frac{12\ \text{mEq} \times 15\ \text{mL}}{20\ \text{mEq}} = 9\ \text{mL}$$

Test-Taking Strategy: Focus on the data in the question, and then follow the formula for the calculation of the correct dose. Verify your answer using a calculator. Once you have determined that 9 mL is the correct amount, look for this measure on the medication cup. Review medication calculation problems if you had difficulty with this question.

Level of Cognitive Ability: Application
Client Needs: Physiological Integrity
Integrated Process: Nursing Process/Implementation
Content Area: Pharmacological and Parenteral Therapies

References
Kee J, Marshall S: *Clinical calculations: with applications to general and specialty areas,* ed 5, Philadelphia, 2004, Saunders, p 80.
Macklin D, Chernecky C, Infortuna H: *Math for clinical practice,* St Louis, 2005, Mosby, p 586.

Multiple Response

238. Which of the following are manifestations of the prodromal stage of inhalation anthrax? Select all that apply.

❑ **1** Fever
❑ **2** Headache
❑ **3** Sore throat
❑ **4** Watery eyes
❑ **5** Mild chest pain
❑ **6** Dry harsh cough

Answer: 1, 5, 6

Rationale: Inhalation anthrax is a bacterial infection caused by the gram-positive, rod-shaped organism *Bacillus anthracis*. Inhalation anthrax is a two-stage illness, and manifestations may not begin until as long as 8 weeks after exposure to the organism. The first stage is the prodromal stage, and the second stage is the fulminant (late) stage. In the prodromal stage manifestations are nonspecific and sometimes difficult to differentiate from influenza or other respiratory disorders. These include fever, fatigue, mild chest pain, and a dry harsh cough. Inhalation anthrax is not accompanied by upper respiratory tract manifestations such as rhinitis, headache, watery eyes, or sore throat. The fulminant stage begins after the client feels a little better and usually begins with sudden onset of breathlessness that rapidly progresses to severe respiratory distress, dyspnea, diaphoresis, stridor on inhalation and exhalation, cyanosis, and high fever. As the disease spreads, the client develops septic shock and meningitis, leading to death within 24 to 36 hours, even if antibiotics are initiated.

Test-Taking Strategy: Specific knowledge regarding the stages of inhalation anthrax and their associated manifestations is needed to answer this question. Remember that inhalation anthrax is not accompanied by upper respiratory tract manifestations of rhinitis, headache, watery eyes, or sore throat. This will assist in answering questions similar to this one. Review the manifestations associated with inhalation anthrax if you had difficulty with this question.

Level of Cognitive Ability: Analysis
Client Needs: Physiological Integrity
Integrated Process: Nursing Process/Assessment
Content Area: Physiological Adaptation

Reference
Ignatavicius D, Workman M: *Medical surgical nursing: critical thinking for collaborative care*, ed 5, Philadelphia, 2006, Saunders, pp 645-646.

Fill-in-the-Blank

239. A nurse is preparing medication for administration to a child and needs to convert the child's weight from pounds (lb) to kilograms (kg). The nurse determines that the child, whose weight is 12.5 lb, weighs how many kilograms? (Round answer to the nearest tenth.)

Answer: _____ **kg**

Answer: 5.7

Rationale: One kg is equal to 2.2 lb. To convert pounds to kilograms, divide the weight in pounds by 2.2 (12.5 lb ÷ 2.2 = 5.68, or 5.7 kg).

Test-Taking Strategy: Use the formula for converting pounds to kilograms, remembering that 1 kg equals 2.2 lb. Verify the answer using a calculator, and remember to round the answer to the nearest tenth. Review this formula if you had difficulty with this question.

Level of Cognitive Ability: Analysis
Client Needs: Physiological Integrity
Integrated Process: Nursing Process/Assessment
Content Area: Pharmacological and Parenteral Therapies

Reference
Kee J, Marshall S: *Clinical calculations: with applications to general and specialty areas,* ed 5, Philadelphia, 2004, Saunders, p 235.

Multiple Response

240. The nurse instructs a mother about measures to prevent parasitic infections in her children. The nurse includes which of the following in the instructions? Select all that apply.

❑ **1** Leave sandboxes uncovered when not in use.

❑ **2** Wash all fruits and vegetables before eating them.

❑ **3** Discourage children from scratching their anal area with bare hands.

❑ **4** Avoid swimming facilities that allow diapered children in the water.

❑ **5** Discourage children from placing their hands in the mouth and biting their nails.

❑ **6** Hand washing with soap and water should be done before eating or handling food and after using the toilet.

Answer: 2, 3, 4, 5, 6

Rationale: Measures that will assist in preventing parasitic infections include washing hands (including under the fingernails) with soap and water before eating or handling food and after using the toilet; discouraging children from placing hands in the mouth and nail biting; discouraging children from scratching the anal area with bare hands; keeping dogs and cats at a distance from play areas; covering sandboxes when not in use; wearing shoes outside; changing diapers frequently and disposing of them properly; avoiding swimming facilities that allow diapered children in the water; and drinking bottled water during camping outings.

Test-Taking Strategy: Focus on the subject, measures to prevent parasitic infections. Read each option carefully, thinking about this subject. Noting the word *uncovered* in option 1 will assist in eliminating this option. Review measures to prevent parasitic infections if you had difficulty with this question.

Level of Cognitive Ability: Application
Client Needs: Safe and Effective Care Environment
Integrated Process: Teaching and Learning
Content Area: Safety and Infection Control

Reference

McKinney E, James S, Murray S, et al: *Maternal-child nursing,* ed 2, Philadelphia, 2005, Saunders, p 1039.

Multiple Response

241. An infant is diagnosed with hypertrophic pyloric stenosis. The nurse reviews the infant's record, expecting to note documentation of which manifestations associated with this condition? Select all that apply.

- ❑ **1** Constipation
- ❑ **2** Bloody mucus (currant jelly) stool
- ❑ **3** Progressive projectile nonbilious vomiting
- ❑ **4** Pelletlike or ribbonlike stools that are foul smelling
- ❑ **5** A movable, palpable, firm olive-shaped mass felt in the right upper quadrant
- ❑ **6** Deep gastric peristaltic waves from the left upper quadrant to right upper quadrant visible immediately before vomiting

Answer: 3, 5, 6

Rationale: Pyloric stenosis results when the circular area of muscle surrounding the pylorus hypertrophies and obstructs gastric emptying. Progressive projectile nonbilious vomiting is a major manifestation of pyloric stenosis. A movable, palpable, firm olive-shaped mass is felt in the right upper quadrant. Deep gastric peristaltic waves from the left upper quadrant to right upper quadrant may be visible immediately before vomiting. Passage of bloody mucus (currant jelly) stool is a manifestation of intussusception. Pelletlike or ribbonlike stools that are foul smelling and chronic constipation are manifestations of Hirschsprung's disease.

Test-Taking Strategy: Focus on the diagnosis. Recall that pyloric stenosis results when the circular area of muscle surrounding the pylorus hypertrophies and obstructs gastric emptying. This will assist in eliminating options 1, 2, and 4 because these manifestations address the lower intestinal tract. Review the manifestations of hypertrophic pyloric stenosis if you had difficulty with this question.

Level of Cognitive Ability: Analysis
Client Needs: Physiological Integrity
Integrated Process: Nursing Process/Assessment
Content Area: Physiological Adaptation

Reference
McKinney E, James S, Murray S, et al: *Maternal-child nursing,* ed 2, Philadelphia, 2005, Saunders, pp 1137, 1140, 1143.

Multiple Response

242. The nurse prepares to administer a dose of digoxin (Lanoxin), checks the client's apical pulse rate, and notes that it is 58 beats/min. The nurse should take which actions? Select all that apply.

- ❏ **1** Assess the client for signs of digoxin toxicity.
- ❏ **2** Notify the physician of the client's apical pulse rate.
- ❏ **3** Check the result of the client's most recent digoxin level.
- ❏ **4** Check the result of the client's most recent potassium level.
- ❏ **5** Give the digoxin and recheck the apical pulse rate in 1 hour.
- ❏ **6** Check the client's blood pressure and administer the digoxin if it is within normal range.

Answer: 1, 2, 3, 4

Rationale: Digoxin is a cardiac glycoside that is used to manage and treat heart failure, control ventricular rate in clients with atrial fibrillation, and treat and prevent recurrent paroxysmal atrial tachycardia. Toxicity can occur as a result of taking this medication, and the nurse always checks the client's apical pulse rate for 1 minute before administering the medication. If the pulse rate is less than 60 beats/min, the medication is withheld and the physician notified. A slowed pulse could be an indication of toxicity; the nurse assesses the client for other signs of digoxin toxicity. The nurse also checks the result of the client's most recent digoxin level (therapeutic level is 0.8 to 2 ng/mL) and the most recent potassium level (normal is 3.5 to 5.1 mEq/L). Hypokalemia predisposes the client to digoxin toxicity.

Test-Taking Strategy: Focus on the data in the question. Recalling that digoxin is withheld for an apical pulse rate less than 60 beats/min will assist in eliminating options 5 and 6. Review nursing implications related to administering digoxin if you had difficulty with this question.

Level of Cognitive Ability: Application
Client Needs: Physiological Integrity
Integrated Process: Nursing Process/Implementation
Content Area: Pharmacological and Parenteral Therapies

Reference
Hodgson B, Kizior R: *Saunders nursing drug handbook 2007*, Philadelphia, 2007, Saunders, p 358.

Multiple Response

243. Furosemide (Lasix) is prescribed for a client, and the nurse instructs the client about the medication. Which instructions should the nurse provide to the client? Select all that apply.

- ❏ **1** Restrict fluid intake.
- ❏ **2** Expect some muscle weakness.
- ❏ **3** Take the medication at bedtime.
- ❏ **4** Expect increased urinary output.
- ❏ **5** Eat foods that are high in potassium.
- ❏ **6** Expect to experience some ringing in the ears.

Answer: 4, 5

Rationale: Furosemide is a loop diuretic. The client is instructed to take the medication in the morning and with food if gastrointestinal upset occurs and to expect increased frequency and volume of urination. The client is also instructed to eat foods high in potassium because of the risk for hypokalemia. The client is also instructed to monitor for signs of hypokalemia, including muscle weakness; if this occurs, the physician is notified. Ototoxicity is also an adverse effect, and the client is instructed to contact the physician if ringing in the ears occurs. Fluid intake should not be restricted; the client should be instructed to maintain a normal intake unless otherwise prescribed.

Test-Taking Strategy: Focus on the name of the medication and recall that furosemide is a loop diuretic that is potassium losing. This will assist in determining that options 4 and 5 are correct and that option 3 is incorrect. Next eliminate option 1 because of the word *restrict*. Finally, recalling that hypokalemia and ototoxicity are adverse effects will assist in eliminating options 2 and 6. Review client instructions related to furosemide if you had difficulty with this question.

Level of Cognitive Ability: Application
Client Needs: Physiological Integrity
Integrated Process: Teaching and Learning
Content Area: Pharmacological and Parenteral Therapies

Reference
Hodgson B, Kizior R: *Saunders nursing drug handbook 2007,* Philadelphia, 2007, Saunders, p 525.

Multiple Response

244. Sublingual nitroglycerin tablets have been prescribed for a client to treat episodes of acute angina pectoris. Which instructions should the nurse provide to the client about the medication? Select all that apply.

❏ **1** Take a tablet at the first sign of chest pain.

❏ **2** Take the medication while sitting or lying down.

❏ **3** Check the expiration date on the medication bottle.

❏ **4** Swallow the tablet for the most effective and rapid effect.

❏ **5** Keep the bottle of medication away from heat and moisture.

❏ **6** If the pain is not relieved 5 minutes after taking the tablet, take a second one.

Answer: 1, 2, 3, 5, 6

Rationale: Nitroglycerin is an antianginal and coronary vasodilator. Sublingual nitroglycerin tablets are allowed to dissolve under the tongue (not swallowed), and one is taken at the first sign of chest pain. If the pain is not relieved in 5 minutes, another tablet is taken. A third tablet is taken in 5 minutes if there is no relief from the second one. If pain is still unrelieved, the client should contact the physician or immediately go to the emergency department. The client should take the medication while sitting or lying down because of the risk of hypotension. The client should check the expiration date on the medication bottle and keep the medication away from sources of heat or moisture, since these will affect their effectiveness.

Test-Taking Strategy: Focus on the name of the medication. Recalling that nitroglycerin is an antianginal and coronary vasodilator will assist in selecting the correct options. Also, noting the strategic word *sublingual* in the question will assist in eliminating option 4. Review client instructions for nitroglycerin if you had difficulty with this question.

Level of Cognitive Ability: Application
Client Needs: Physiological Integrity
Integrated Process: Teaching and Learning
Content Area: Pharmacological and Parenteral Therapies

Reference
Hodgson B, Kizior R: *Saunders nursing drug handbook 2007*, Philadelphia, 2007, Saunders, p 845.

Multiple Response

245. Phenytoin (Dilantin) capsules are prescribed for a client in the management of tonic-clonic seizures. The nurse provides which instructions to the client about the medication? Select all that apply.

- ❏ 1 Perform good oral hygiene and gum massage.
- ❏ 2 Plan to have a complete blood cell count drawn monthly.
- ❏ 3 Report signs of infection such as a fever to the physician.
- ❏ 4 Contact the physician if a red-brown discoloration of the urine occurs.
- ❏ 5 Expect some drowsiness initially that diminishes with continued therapy.
- ❏ 6 Break the capsules and sprinkle the granules in apple sauce before taking the medication.

Answer: 1, 2, 3, 5

Rationale: Phenytoin is an anticonvulsant. The client is instructed not to chew or break the capsules and to take the medication with food if gastrointestinal discomfort occurs. Adverse effects include blood dyscrasias. Therefore the client should plan to have a complete blood cell count drawn monthly until a maintenance dose is established and to report signs of infection such as a fever or a sore throat to the physician. Gingival hyperplasia can also occur, and the client is instructed to perform good oral hygiene and gum massage and schedule regular dental visits. A red-brown discoloration of the urine is a harmless side effect, and drowsiness diminishes with continued therapy.

Test-Taking Strategy: Use general medication guidelines to assist in determining that option 6 is incorrect. Capsules should not be broken or chewed. Next it is necessary to know that a red-brown discoloration of the urine is a harmless side effect. Remember that gingival hyperplasia, blood dyscrasias, and drowsiness can occur with this medication. Review client instructions related to phenytoin if you had difficulty with this question.

Level of Cognitive Ability: Application
Client Needs: Physiological Integrity
Integrated Process: Teaching and Learning
Content Area: Pharmacological and Parenteral Therapies

Reference
Hodgson B, Kizior R: *Saunders nursing drug handbook 2007,* Philadelphia, 2007, Saunders, p 930.

Figure/Illustration with a Fill-in-the-Blank

246. A client sustained a burn injury and experienced burns to the anterior upper legs, anterior thorax, and perineum. According to the rule of nines, what percentage of the total body surface area (TBSA) sustained a burn injury? (Refer to figure.)

Answer: _____ %

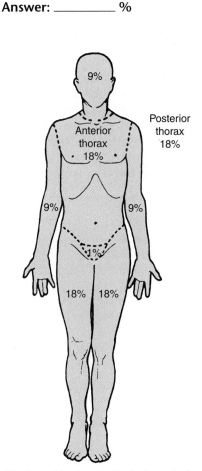

From Black J, Hawks J: *Medical-surgical nursing: clinical management for positive outcomes,* ed 7, Philadelphia, 2005, Saunders.

Answer: 28

Rationale: The rule of nines provides a quick method for estimating the extent of a burn injury in the adult. The basis of the rule is that the body is divided into anatomic sections, each of which represents 9% or a multiple of 9% of the TBSA. Therefore, if the anterior upper legs (9%, with 4.5% for each anterior upper leg), anterior thorax (18%), and perineum (1%) are burned, the total is 28%.

Test-Taking Strategy: Focus on the data in the question and note the strategic words *anterior upper legs, anterior thorax, and perineum.* Next focus on the figure and use mathematics to determine the total percent. Review the rule of nines if you had difficulty with this question.

Level of Cognitive Ability: Analysis
Client Needs: Physiological Integrity
Integrated Process: Nursing Process/Assessment
Content Area: Physiological Adaptation

Reference
Black J, Hawks J: *Medical-surgical nursing: clinical management for positive outcomes,* ed 7, Philadelphia, 2005, Saunders, pp 1442-1443.

Prioritizing (Ordered Response)

247. Identify the steps in order of priority for performing an electrocardiogram (ECG). (Number 1 is the first step and number 6 is the last step.)

____ Wash hands.
____ Clean the gel from the client's skin.
____ Apply conductive gel to the client's skin.
____ Disconnect the electrodes from the client.
____ Attach electrodes to the client's skin and obtain a reading.
____ Explain the importance of lying still, breathing normally, and refraining from talking during the test.

Answer: 1, 6, 3, 5, 4, 2

Rationale: The ECG is a noninvasive tool for evaluating the heart rhythm and displays the electrical activity of the heart. The nurse first washes the hands and then explains the procedure to the client, including the importance of lying still, breathing normally, and refraining from talking during the test. The nurse next applies conductive gel to the client's skin, attaches electrodes to the client's skin, and adjusts the monitor to obtain a reading. Once the reading is obtained, the nurse disconnects the electrodes from the client and cleans the gel from the client's skin.

Test-Taking Strategy: Visualize this procedure to answer correctly. Remember that the nurse washes his or her hands first and then explains the procedure to the client. Review this procedure if you had difficulty with this question.

Level of Cognitive Ability: Application
Client Needs: Physiological Integrity
Integrated Process: Nursing Process/Implementation
Content Area: Physiological Adaptation

Reference

Black J, Hawks J: *Medical-surgical nursing: clinical management for positive outcomes,* ed 7, Philadelphia, 2005, Saunders, p 1582.

Figure/Illustration with a Multiple Choice

248. The nurse is performing a neurological assessment. The nurse tests the function of which reflex by performing this assessment action? (Refer to figure.)

❑ 1 Biceps
❑ 2 Patellar
❑ 3 Achilles
❑ 4 Brachioradialis

From Ignatavicius D, Workman M: *Medical surgical nursing: critical thinking for collaborative care,* ed 5, Philadelphia, 2006, Saunders.

Answer: 1

Rationale: The biceps reflex is tested at the biceps tendon in the antecubital fossa. The patellar reflex is tested over the patellar tendon just below the patella. The Achilles reflex is tested at the Achilles tendon at the level of the ankle malleolus. The brachioradialis reflex is tested at the brachioradialis tendon located directly about 1 to 2 inches (2.5 to 5 cm) above the wrist.

Test-Taking Strategy: Focus on the figure. Using knowledge of anatomy and the location of tendons will direct you to option 1. Review this assessment technique if you had difficulty with this question.

Level of Cognitive Ability: Application
Client Needs: Health Promotion and Maintenance
Integrated Process: Nursing Process/Assessment
Content Area: Prevention and Detection of Health Alterations

References
Ignatavicius D, Workman M: *Medical surgical nursing: critical thinking for collaborative care,* ed 5, Philadelphia, 2006, Saunders, p 937.
Wilson S, Giddens J: *Health assessment for nursing practice,* ed 3, St Louis, 2005, Mosby, p 630.

Multiple Response

249. Hepatitis A is transmitted by which of the following methods? Select all that apply.

❑ **1** Drinking contaminated water
❑ **2** Eating shellfish caught in contaminated water
❑ **3** Abusing drugs and using a contaminated needle
❑ **4** Coming into blood contact with an infected person
❑ **5** Transferring from an infected mother to the child at birth
❑ **6** Eating food contaminated by food handlers infected with HAV

Answer: 1, 2, 6

Rationale: The causative agent of hepatitis A, hepatitis A virus (HAV), is a ribonucleic acid virus of the enterovirus family. It is spread via the fecal-oral route by the oral ingestion of fecal contaminants. Sources of infection include contaminated water, shellfish caught in contaminated water, and food contaminated by food handlers infected with HAV. The virus may also be spread by oral-anal sexual activity. Hepatitis B is transmitted by blood contact with an infected person, by drug abuse and use of a contaminated needle, and from an infected mother to the child at birth.

Test-Taking Strategy: Focus on the subject, transmission routes of hepatitis A. Recalling that HAV is spread via the fecal-oral route by the oral ingestion of fecal contaminants will direct you to the correct options. Review the routes of transmission of the various types of hepatitis if you had difficulty with this question.

Level of Cognitive Ability: Analysis
Client Needs: Safe and Effective Care Environment
Integrated Process: Nursing Process/Assessment
Content Area: Safety and Infection Control

Reference
Ignatavicius D, Workman M: *Medical surgical nursing: critical thinking for collaborative care,* ed 5, Philadelphia, 2006, Saunders, pp 1382-1383.

Multiple Response

250. A nurse caring for a client receiving mechanical ventilation via an oral endotracheal tube understands that the causes of the high-pressure alarm sounding include which of the following? Select all that apply.

- ❑ **1** A kink in the tube
- ❑ **2** The client fighting the ventilator
- ❑ **3** Increased secretions in the airway
- ❑ **4** A cuff leak in the endotracheal tube
- ❑ **5** The client biting on the endotracheal tube
- ❑ **6** The ventilator tubing disconnecting from the endotracheal tube

Answer: 1, 2, 3, 5

Rationale: The high-pressure alarm sounds when the peak inspiratory pressure reaches the set alarm limit. Causes include an increased amount of secretions in the airways or a mucus plug; the client coughing, gagging, or biting on the oral endotracheal tube; the client being anxious or fighting the ventilator; decreased airway size related to wheezing or bronchospasm; pneumothorax; displacement of the artificial airway and the endotracheal tube slipping into the right mainstem bronchus; or obstruction of the endotracheal tube because of the client lying on the tube or water or a kink in the tubing. The low-pressure alarm sounds when there is a leak or disconnection in the ventilator circuit or a leak in the client's artificial airway cuff.

Test-Taking Strategy: Note the strategic words *high-pressure alarm*. Recalling that the high-pressure alarm sounds when the peak inspiratory pressure reaches the set alarm limit assists in eliminating options 4 and 6. Review the causes of ventilator alarms if you had difficulty with this question.

Level of Cognitive Ability: Analysis
Client Needs: Physiological Integrity
Integrated Process: Nursing Process/Evaluation
Content Area: Reduction of Risk Potential

Reference
Ignatavicius D, Workman M: *Medical surgical nursing: critical thinking for collaborative care,* ed 5, Philadelphia, 2006, Saunders, p 667.

Multiple Response

251. The nurse provides home care instructions to the mother of a newborn infant requiring phototherapy. Which instructions does the nurse provide? Select all that apply.

❑ **1** Feed the infant every 2 to 3 hours.
❑ **2** Count the infant's wet diapers and stools.
❑ **3** Ensure that the infant receives phototherapy 24 hours a day.
❑ **4** Check the infant's axillary temperature before every feeding.
❑ **5** Dress the infant in a diaper to expose as much skin as possible to the lights.
❑ **6** Close the infant's eyes and place patches over the eyes before positioning the infant under the lights.

Answer: 1, 2, 4, 5, 6

Rationale: Phototherapy, in which special lights are placed over the infant, is used in the treatment of jaundice. The infant is dressed only in a diaper to expose as much skin as possible to the lights and is positioned under the lights at the proper distance according to manufacturer's instructions. Placing the lights too close to the infant can result in burns; placing the lights too far away results in ineffective treatment. The infant's eyes are closed and patches are placed over the eyes before positioning the infant under the lights; the patches are checked every hour. The infant may be removed from the phototherapy for feedings, diaper changes, and other care but should receive phototherapy for 18 hours a day. The infant's axillary temperature is checked before every feeding and should remain between 97.7° and 99.5° F. The infant is fed every 2 to 3 hours because the phototherapy causes the infant to lose fluid from the skin and have loose stools, leading to dehydration. The mother should count the infant's wet diapers and stools and increase feedings if the infant has less than six wet diapers a day or if the urine appears dark.

Test-Taking Strategy: Think about the purpose of phototherapy and visualize each option, keeping in mind that safety and prevention of dehydration are primary concerns. Noting the words *24 hours a day* in option 3 will assist in eliminating this option. Review care of the infant receiving phototherapy if you had difficulty with this question.

Level of Cognitive Ability: Application
Client Needs: Physiological Integrity
Integrated Process: Teaching and Learning
Content Area: Reduction of Risk Potential

Reference
McKinney E, James S, Murray S, et al: *Maternal-child nursing,* ed 2, Philadelphia, 2005, Saunders, p 751.

Multiple Response

252. The nurse provides dietary instructions to a client who has a vitamin B_{12} deficiency. The nurse tells the client that which foods are high in vitamin B_{12}? Select all that apply.

- ❑ **1** Liver
- ❑ **2** Nuts
- ❑ **3** Raisins
- ❑ **4** Oranges
- ❑ **5** Mushrooms
- ❑ **6** Dried beans

Answer: 1, 2, 4, 6

Rationale: Foods high in vitamin B_{12} include liver, organ meats, dried beans, nuts, green leafy vegetables, citrus fruits, and brewer's yeast. Raisins are high in iron. Mushrooms are high in potassium.

Test-Taking Strategy: Specific knowledge regarding the foods high in vitamin B_{12} is needed to answer this question. Remember that foods high in vitamin B_{12} include liver, organ meats, dried beans, nuts, green leafy vegetables, citrus fruits, and brewer's yeast. Review the foods high in vitamin B_{12} if you had difficulty with this question.

Level of Cognitive Ability: Application
Client Needs: Physiological Integrity
Integrated Process: Teaching and Learning
Content Area: Basic Care and Comfort

Reference

Ignatavicius D, Workman M: *Medical surgical nursing: critical thinking for collaborative care,* ed 5, Philadelphia, 2006, Saunders, p 894.

Multiple Response

253. Identify the immediate interventions for a client experiencing autonomic dysreflexia. Select all that apply.

❏ **1** Notify the physician.
❏ **2** Loosen tight clothing.
❏ **3** Check the client for fecal impaction.
❏ **4** Place a fan on the client to cool the client.
❏ **5** Check the Foley catheter for kinks or obstructions.
❏ **6** Place the client in a modified Trendelenburg's position.

Answer: 1, 2, 3, 5

Rationale: Autonomic dysreflexia is characterized by a cluster of clinical manifestations that result when multiple spinal cord autonomic responses discharge simultaneously. The manifestations result from an exaggerated sympathetic response to a noxious stimuli below the level of the cord lesion. Manifestations include a sudden severe throbbing headache, severe hypertension, bradycardia, flushing above the level of the lesion (face and chest), nasal stuffiness, sweating, nausea, blurred vision, piloerection, and apprehension. If the client experiences autonomic dysreflexia, the nurse places the client in a sitting position; notifies the physician; loosens tight clothing on the client; assesses and treats the cause; checks the Foley catheter for kinks or obstructions or, if a Foley catheter is not present, checks for bladder distention; checks the client for fecal impaction; checks the room temperature to ensure that it is not too cool or drafty; monitors the blood pressure every 10 to 15 minutes; and administers medication as prescribed.

Test-Taking Strategy: Think about the pathophysiology of autonomic dysreflexia. Recalling that it results from an exaggerated sympathetic response will assist in eliminating option 4. Recalling that severe hypertension occurs will assist in eliminating option 6. Review care for the client experiencing autonomic dysreflexia if you had difficulty with this question.

Level of Cognitive Ability: Application
Client Needs: Physiological Integrity
Integrated Process: Nursing Process/Implementation
Content Area: Physiological Adaptation

Reference
Ignatavicius D, Workman M: *Medical surgical nursing: critical thinking for collaborative care,* ed 5, Philadelphia, 2006, Saunders, p 988.

Multiple Response

254. What nursing interventions should the nurse take when working with parents who experienced the death of their fetus? Select all that apply.

❑ **1** Encourage the parents to avoid viewing the fetus.
❑ **2** Refer the parents to appropriate community support groups.
❑ **3** Clean and wrap the fetus in a clean blanket for parental viewing.
❑ **4** Identify the parents' perceptions and feelings about the fetal death.
❑ **5** Inform the parents that spiritual support such as baptism or a memorial service is not important.
❑ **6** Provide the parents with a certificate that indicates vital statistics, along with identification bands, locks of hair, and footprints.

Answer: 2, 3, 4, 6

Rationale: Allowing the parents quiet time to hold and view the fetus and preparing the fetus for viewing by cleansing the body and wrapping the fetus in a clean blanket help the parents realize the reality of the loss and provide a supportive setting for grieving. The nurse should identify the parents' perceptions and feelings about the fetal death to correct any misconceptions and alleviate guilt. Providing a certificate that indicates vital statistics, along with identification bands, locks of hair, and footprints, also lends reality to the situation and supports the grieving process. Providing spiritual support as needed, such as baptism or a memorial service, assists with moving through the grieving process. Appropriate community support groups can facilitate grieving with group input and shared experiences.

Test-Taking Strategy: Focus on the parents' feelings and recall interventions that are appropriate as they move through the grieving process. Eliminate option 1 because of the word *avoid* and option 5 because of the words *not important.* Review interventions to support the grieving process if you had difficulty with this question.

Level of Cognitive Ability: Application
Client Needs: Psychosocial Integrity
Integrated Process: Nursing Process/Implementation
Content Area: Psychosocial Adaptation

Reference
Lowdermilk D, Perry S: *Maternity and women's health care,* ed 8, St Louis, 2004, Mosby, p 1165.

Multiple Response

255. The nurse monitors a client receiving intravenous therapy for signs of complications. Which of the following are manifestations of an air embolism? Select all that apply.

- ❑ **1** Dyspnea
- ❑ **2** Chest pain
- ❑ **3** Bradycardia
- ❑ **4** Hypertension
- ❑ **5** Lightheadedness
- ❑ **6** Loud churning sound heard over the pericardium on auscultation

Answer: 1, 2, 5, 6

Rationale: An air embolism occurs when air enters the central venous system during catheter insertion, tubing changes, catheter rupture, and catheter removal. Manifestations include chest pain, dyspnea, hypoxia, anxiety, tachycardia, hypotension, nausea, lightheadedness, and dizziness. A loud churning sound may be heard over the pericardium on auscultation.

Test-Taking Strategy: Focus on the subject, the manifestations of an air embolism. Thinking about the pathophysiology and the cause of an air embolism will assist in answering correctly. Remember that tachycardia and hypotension occur in this complication. Review the manifestations of an air embolism if you had difficulty with this question.

Level of Cognitive Ability: Analysis
Client Needs: Physiological Integrity
Integrated Process: Nursing Process/Assessment
Content Area: Pharmacological and Parenteral Therapies

Reference
Ignatavicius D, Workman M: *Medical surgical nursing: critical thinking for collaborative care,* ed 5, Philadelphia, 2006, Saunders, p 263.

Multiple Response

256. The nurse conducts an interview and collects data regarding the client's health and health history. What statements are appropriate for the nurse to document? Select all that apply.

❏ 1 The client appears irritable.
❏ 2 The client takes a daily multivitamin.
❏ 3 The client has a history of depressive episodes.
❏ 4 The client has a family history of hypertension.
❏ 5 The client had an appendectomy at the age of 30 years.
❏ 6 The client is apparently having a bad day and responds abruptly to questions asked.

Answer: 2, 3, 4, 5

Rationale: During the health history the nurse communicates with the client and collects information about the client's current state of health, previous illnesses and surgeries, and family history. Complete, accurate, and descriptive data need to be documented. When documenting, the nurse avoids statements that express value judgments about the client such as "the client appears irritable" or "the client is apparently having a bad day and responds abruptly to questions asked."

Test-Taking Strategy: Read each option carefully. Recalling that guidelines related to documentation include complete, accurate, and descriptive data will assist in determining that options 1 and 6 are inappropriate to document. Review guidelines for documentation if you had difficulty with this question.

Level of Cognitive Ability: Application
Client Needs: Safe and Effective Care Environment
Integrated Process: Communication and Documentation
Content Area: Management of Care

Reference
Wilson S, Giddens J: *Health assessment for nursing practice,* ed 3, St Louis, 2005, Mosby, pp 2, 39.

Fill-in-the-Blank

257. A physician's order reads morphine sulfate gr $^1/_6$ intramuscular stat. The medication ampule reads morphine sulfate 10 mg/mL. A nurse prepares how many milliliters to administer the correct dose?

Answer: _____ mL

Answer: 1

Rationale: It is necessary to convert gr $^1/_6$ to milligrams, then use the formula to calculate the correct dose.

Conversion

60 mg : gr 1 :: x mg : gr $^1/_6$

$$1x = \frac{1}{6} \times \frac{60}{1}$$

$$x = \frac{60}{6} = 10 \text{ mg}$$

Formula

$$\frac{\text{Desired} \times \text{mL}}{\text{Available}} = \text{mL per dose}$$

$$\frac{10 \text{ mg} \times 1 \text{ mL}}{10 \text{ mg}} = 1 \text{ mL}$$

Test-Taking Strategy: In this medication calculation problem, it is necessary to first convert grains to milligrams. Next, follow the formula for calculating the correct dose. Use a calculator to verify the answer. Review medication calculation problems if you had difficulty with this question.

Level of Cognitive Ability: Application
Client Needs: Physiological Integrity
Integrated Process: Nursing Process/Implementation
Content Area: Pharmacological and Parenteral Therapies

Reference

Kee J, Marshall S: *Clinical calculations: with applications to general and specialty areas,* ed 5, Philadelphia, 2004, Saunders, pp 35, 80.

Prioritizing (Ordered Response)

258. List in order of priority the steps of the teaching process for a client who needs to learn about a low-fat diet. (Number 1 is the first step and number 6 is the last step.)

___ Implement the teaching plan.

___ Determine the client's learning needs.

___ Collect data on the client's knowledge of low-fat foods.

___ Evaluate client learning about low-fat foods on the basis of achieving objectives

___ Make an educational diagnosis such as "Deficient Knowledge about the foods that are low in fat."

___ Prepare a teaching plan that includes objectives, content, time frame, teaching format, and teaching aids.

Answer: 5, 2, 1, 6, 3, 4

Rationale: In the teaching-learning process the nurse would first collect and analyze data about the client's knowledge and then identify the client's learning needs. Next the nurse would identify an educational diagnosis, prepare a teaching plan, and then implement the plan. Finally, the nurse evaluates client learning on the basis of objectives and reassesses learning needs.

Test-Taking Strategy: Focus on the subject, the steps that you would take in teaching a client about a low-fat diet. If you can recall the steps of the nursing process and remember that these steps progress in a systematic order—assessment, analysis, planning, implementation, evaluation—you will be able to determine the steps in the teaching-learning process. Review the steps of the teaching-learning process if you had difficulty with this question.

Level of Cognitive Ability: Application
Client Needs: Health Promotion and Maintenance
Integrated Process: Teaching and Learning
Content Area: Prevention and Detection of Health Alterations

Reference
Harkreader H, Hogan MA: *Fundamentals of nursing: caring and clinical judgment,* ed 2, Philadelphia, 2004, Saunders, p 261.

Fill-in-the-Blank

259. A physician's order reads levothyroxine (Synthroid), 100 mcg orally daily. The medication label reads levothyroxine, 0.1 mg per tablet. A nurse administers how many tablet(s) to the client?

Answer: ＿＿＿＿＿ **tablet(s)**

Answer: 1

Rationale: It is necessary to convert 100 mcg to milligrams. In the metric system, to convert smaller to larger, divide by 1000 or move the decimal 3 places to the left. Therefore, 100 mcg = 0.1 mg. The nurse would administer 1 tablet.

Test-Taking Strategy: Focus on the data in the question. In this medication calculation problem, it is necessary to first convert micrograms to milligrams. Since 100 mcg = 0.1 mg, the nurse would administer 1 tablet. Review medication calculation problems if you had difficulty with this question.

Level of Cognitive Ability: Application
Client Needs: Physiological Integrity
Integrated Process: Nursing Process/Implementation
Content Area: Pharmacological and Parenteral Therapies

Reference

Kee J, Marshall S: *Clinical calculations: with applications to general and specialty areas,* ed 5, Philadelphia, 2004, Saunders, pp 35, 80.

Multiple Response

260. The nurse is assessing a client with angina pectoris. Which of the following are characteristics of the substernal chest pain that occurs with this condition? Select all that apply.

❑ **1** Occurs without cause
❑ **2** Radiates to the left arm
❑ **3** Lasts less than 15 minutes
❑ **4** Usually occurs in the morning
❑ **5** Is relieved by rest or nitroglycerin
❑ **6** Is precipitated by exertion or stress

Answer: 2, 3, 5, 6

Rationale: Angina pectoris is a temporary imbalance between the coronary artery's ability to supply oxygen and the cardiac muscle's demand for oxygen. The substernal chest pain that occurs in angina radiates to the left arm, is precipitated by exertion or stress, is relieved by rest or nitroglycerin, and lasts less than 15 minutes. Myocardial infarction occurs when myocardial tissue is abruptly and severely deprived of oxygen. The substernal chest pain that occurs in myocardial infarction radiates to the left arm, back, or jaw; occurs without cause, usually in the morning; is relieved only by opioids; and lasts 30 minutes or longer. The client with myocardial infarction also experiences nausea, diaphoresis, dyspnea, dysrhythmias, epigastric distress, and fatigue.

Test-Taking Strategy: Focus on the subject, the characteristics of the substernal chest pain that occurs with angina pectoris. Remember that the pain that occurs in angina radiates to the left arm, is precipitated by exertion or stress, is relieved by rest or nitroglycerin, and lasts less than 15 minutes. Review the characteristics of the pain in angina pectoris if you had difficulty with this question.

Level of Cognitive Ability: Analysis
Client Needs: Physiological Integrity
Integrated Process: Nursing Process/Assessment
Content Area: Physiological Adaptation

Reference
Ignatavicius D, Workman M: *Medical surgical nursing: critical thinking for collaborative care,* ed 5, Philadelphia, 2006, Saunders, p 845.

Multiple Response

261. A client with kidney failure is at risk for hyperkalemia. The nurse monitors for which of the following clinical manifestations of hyperkalemia? Select all that apply.

- ❏ **1** Muscle twitches
- ❏ **2** Tall T waves on ECG
- ❏ **3** ST depression on ECG
- ❏ **4** Deep tendon hyporeflexia
- ❏ **5** Hyperactive bowel sounds
- ❏ **6** Flat P waves on electrocardiogram (ECG)

Answer: 1, 2, 5, 6

Rationale: Hyperkalemia is a serum potassium level greater than 5.0 mEq/L. Clinical manifestations include ECG abnormalities such as tall T waves, widened QRS complexes, prolonged PR intervals, and flat P waves. Other manifestations include muscle twitches, cramps, and paresthesias; and increased bowel motility, hyperactive bowel sounds, and diarrhea. Deep tendon hyporeflexia and ST depression on ECG are manifestations of hypokalemia.

Test-Taking Strategy: Focus on the subject, manifestations of hyperkalemia. Note that options 1 and 5 are comparative or alike in that they identify an increased, or *hyper,* response; these are manifestations of *hyper*kalemia. Next remember that flat P waves and tall T waves on ECG are manifestations of hyperkalemia. Review the manifestations of hyperkalemia if you had difficulty with this question.

Level of Cognitive Ability: Analysis
Client Needs: Physiological Integrity
Integrated Process: Nursing Process/Assessment
Content Area: Physiological Adaptation

Reference
Ignatavicius D, Workman M: *Medical surgical nursing: critical thinking for collaborative care,* ed 5, Philadelphia, 2006, Saunders, p 232.

Multiple Response

262. The nurse provides dietary instructions to a client who needs to increase his intake of potassium and instructs the client to consume which foods? Select all that apply.

    ❑ 1 Eggs
    ❑ 2 Kiwi
    ❑ 3 Butter
    ❑ 4 Cereal
    ❑ 5 Bananas
    ❑ 6 Oranges

Answer: 2, 5, 6

Rationale: Foods highest in potassium include bananas, cantaloupe, kiwi, oranges, avocados, broccoli, beans, mushrooms, potatoes, and spinach. Foods that are low in potassium include eggs, breads, butter, cereals, apples, apricots, berries, cherries, grapefruit, peaches, pineapple, and cranberries. Vegetables low in potassium include alfalfa sprouts, cabbage, carrots, cauliflower, celery, eggplant, green beans, lettuce, onions, peas, peppers, and squash.

Test-Taking Strategy: Focus on the subject, foods high in potassium. Remember that fruits high in potassium include bananas, cantaloupe, kiwi, and oranges. This will assist in answering questions similar to this one. Review high-potassium foods if you had difficulty with this question.

Level of Cognitive Ability: Application
Client Needs: Physiological Integrity
Integrated Process: Teaching and Learning
Content Area: Physiological Adaptation

Reference

Ignatavicius D, Workman M: *Medical surgical nursing: critical thinking for collaborative care,* ed 5, Philadelphia, 2006, Saunders, p 233.

Multiple Response

263. The nurse provides home care instructions for a client with acquired immunodeficiency syndrome (AIDS) about infection control measures. The nurse includes which of the following in the instructions? Select all that apply.

- ❑ **1** Use only paper plates for eating.
- ❑ **2** Use good hand-washing techniques.
- ❑ **3** Avoid sharing razors or toothbrushes.
- ❑ **4** Clean bathroom surfaces with regular household cleaners weekly.
- ❑ **5** Soak rags, mops, and sponges used for cleaning in a 1:10 solution of household bleach (1 part bleach to 10 parts water) for 5 minutes to disinfect them.
- ❑ **6** Wipe up any vomitus or other body fluid spills with soap and water and disinfect the area with a 1:10 solution of household bleach (1 part bleach to 10 parts water).

Answer: 2, 3, 5, 6

Rationale: Infection control measures for the client with AIDS include measures that prevent the spread of infection through contact with body fluids from the infected individual. Good hand-washing techniques and Standard Precautions are implemented. The client is instructed to avoid sharing razors or toothbrushes or any other items that may cause exposure to body fluids. It is unnecessary to use only paper plates, as long as dishes and eating utensils are washed in hot water and dishwasher soap and detergent. Bathroom surfaces are cleaned with regular household cleaners and then disinfected with a 1:10 solution of household bleach. Rags, mops, and sponges used for cleaning are soaked in a 1:10 solution of household bleach for 5 minutes to disinfect them. Vomitus or other body fluid spills are wiped up with soap and water, and then the area is disinfected with a 1:10 solution of household bleach.

Test-Taking Strategy: Focus on the subject, infection control measures for the client with AIDS. Read each option, keeping in mind which measures will prevent contact with body fluids. This will direct you to the correct options. Review these measures if you had difficulty with this question.

Level of Cognitive Ability: Application
Client Needs: Safe and Effective Care Environment
Integrated Process: Teaching and Learning
Content Area: Safety and Infection Control

Reference
Ignatavicius D, Workman M: *Medical surgical nursing: critical thinking for collaborative care,* ed 5, Philadelphia, 2006, Saunders, p 447.

Multiple Response

264. The nurse instructs a client that which dietary habits will reduce the risk of cancer? Select all that apply.

- ❏ 1 Eating bran
- ❏ 2 Increasing the intake of red meats
- ❏ 3 Eating foods low in vitamin C because of their acidity
- ❏ 4 Eating foods high in vitamin A such as apricots and carrots
- ❏ 5 Eating cruciferous vegetables such as broccoli and Brussels sprouts
- ❏ 6 Avoiding nitrates such as those found in lunch meats, sausage, and bacon

Answer: 1, 4, 5, 6

Rationale: Dietary habits to reduce the risk of cancer include avoiding excessive intake of animal fat; avoiding nitrates such as those found in lunch meats, sausage, and bacon; minimizing the intake of red meats; eating sufficient bran; eating cruciferous vegetables such as broccoli, cabbage, cauliflower, and Brussels sprouts; eating foods high in vitamin A such as apricots, leafy green and yellow vegetables, and carrots; and eating foods high in vitamin C such as fresh fruits and vegetables, especially citrus fruits. Clients are also instructed to minimize alcohol consumption.

Test-Taking Strategy: Focus on the subject, dietary habits that will reduce the risk of cancer. Recalling that high-fiber foods, including fruits and vegetables, are important to consume, and that high-fat foods and foods that contain preservatives such as nitrates need to be avoided, will assist in answering the question. Review these dietary measures if you had difficulty with this question.

Level of Cognitive Ability: Application
Client Needs: Health Promotion and Maintenance
Integrated Process: Teaching and Learning
Content Area: Prevention and Detection of Health Alterations

Reference
Ignatavicius D, Workman M: *Medical surgical nursing: critical thinking for collaborative care,* ed 5, Philadelphia, 2006, Saunders, p 447.

Multiple Response

265. The nurse instructs a client receiving external radiation therapy about skin care. Which statements by the client indicate an understanding of the instructions? Select all that apply.

- ❏ **1** "I can lie in the sun as long as I limit the time to 2 hours daily."
- ❏ **2** "I should wear snug clothing to support the irradiated skin area."
- ❏ **3** "I should wash the irradiated area gently each day with a mild soap and water."
- ❏ **4** "After bathing I should dry the area with a patting motion using a clean soft towel."
- ❏ **5** "I should avoid the use of powders, lotions, or creams on the skin area being irradiated."
- ❏ **6** "I should avoid removing the markings on the skin when bathing until the entire course of radiation is complete."

Answer: 3, 4, 5, 6

Rationale: The purpose of radiation therapy is to destroy cancer cells with minimal exposure of the normal cells to the damaging effects of the radiation. Because external radiation therapy can cause altered skin integrity, special measures need to be taken to protect the skin. These measures include washing the irradiated area gently (using the hand rather than a wash cloth) each day with either water alone or water and a mild soap (rinse soap thoroughly); drying the area with a patting motion (not a rubbing motion) with a clean soft towel; avoiding removing the markings on the skin when bathing until the entire course of radiation is complete because these markings indicate exactly where the beam of radiation is to be focused; avoiding the use of powders, lotions, or creams on the skin area being irradiated unless prescribed by the physician; avoiding wearing clothing or items that bind or rub the irradiated skin area; and avoiding heat exposure or sun exposure to the irradiated area.

Test-Taking Strategy: Note the strategic words, *indicate an understanding of the instructions.* Recall that external radiation therapy can cause altered skin integrity and that special measures need to be taken to protect the skin. Read each option with this in mind to direct you to the correct options. Review these skin care measures if you had difficulty with this question.

Level of Cognitive Ability: Analysis
Client Needs: Physiological Integrity
Integrated Process: Nursing Process/Evaluation
Content Area: Physiological Adaptation

Reference
Ignatavicius D, Workman M: *Medical surgical nursing: critical thinking for collaborative care,* ed 5, Philadelphia, 2006, Saunders, p 491.

REFERENCES

Harkreader H, Hogan MA: *Fundamentals of nursing: caring and clinical judgment,* ed 2, Philadelphia, 2004, Saunders.

Hodgson B, Kizior R: *Saunders nursing drug handbook 2007,* Philadelphia, 2007, Saunders.

Ignatavicius D, Workman M: *Medical surgical nursing: critical thinking for collaborative care,* ed 5, Philadelphia, 2006, Saunders.

Kee J, Marshall S: *Clinical calculations: with applications to general and specialty areas,* ed 5, Philadelphia, 2004, Saunders.

Lowdermilk D, Perry S: *Maternity and women's health care,* ed 8, St Louis, 2004, Mosby.

Macklin D, Chernecky C, Infortuna H: *Math for clinical practice,* St Louis, 2005, Mosby.

McKinney E, James S, Murray S, et al: *Maternal-child nursing,* ed 2, Philadelphia, 2005, Saunders.

Mosby's medical, nursing, and allied health dictionary, ed 7, St Louis, 2006, Mosby.

National Council of State Boards of Nursing: www.ncsbn.org.

National Council of State Boards of Nursing: *National Council of State Boards of Nursing Test Plan for the NCLEX-RN® Examination* (effective date: April 2007), Chicago, 2006, The Council.

Potter P, Perry A: *Fundamentals of nursing,* ed 6, St Louis, 2005, Mosby.

Wilson S, Giddens J: *Health assessment for nursing practice,* ed 3, St Louis, 2005, Mosby.